# Sudden Deaths
# in Custody

# FORENSIC
# SCIENCE AND MEDICINE

*Steven B. Karch, MD,* SERIES EDITOR

# SUDDEN DEATHS
# IN CUSTODY

*Edited by*

## Darrell L. Ross, PhD
*Department of Criminal Justice, East Carolina University, Greenville, NC*

## Theodore C. Chan, MD
*Department of Emergency Medicine, University of California, San Diego, CA*

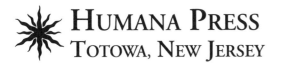
HUMANA PRESS
TOTOWA, NEW JERSEY

© 2006 Humana Press Inc.
999 Riverview Drive, Suite 208
Totowa, New Jersey 07512
**www.humanapress.com**

This publication is printed on acid-free paper. ∞

ANSI Z39.48-1984 (American Standards Institute) Permanence of Paper for Printed Library Materials.

Production editor: Robin B. Weisberg

Cover design by Patricia F. Cleary

For additional copies, pricing for bulk purchases, and/or information about other Humana titles, contact Humana at the above address or at any of the following numbers: Tel.: 973-256-1699; Fax: 973-256-8341; E-mail: orders@humanapr.com; or visit our Website: www.humanapress.com

Printed in the United States of America. 10 9 8 7 6 5 4 3 2 1
E-ISBN 1-59745-015-4
Library of Congress Cataloging-in-Publication Data

Sudden deaths in custody / edited by Darrell L. Ross, Theodore C. Chan.
    p. ; cm. -- (Forensic science and medicine)
  Includes bibliographical references and index.
  ISBN 1-58829-475-7 (alk. paper)
   1. Arrest (Police methods)--Health aspects--United States.
  2. Restraint of prisoners--United States. 3. Prisoners--United
States--Death. 4. Sudden death--United States. 5. Violent deaths
--United States.   I. Ross, Darrell L. (Darrell Lee), 1951-   .
II. Chan, Theodore C. III. Series.
   [DNLM: 1. Death, Sudden--etiology. 2. Restraint, Physical
--adverse effects. 3. Forensic Medicine--methods. 4. Police.
5. Prisoners. 6. Violence.    W 825 S976 2006]
  HV8143.S88 2006
  614'.1--dc22
                                                    2005013427

# Preface

Sudden in-custody restraint deaths have emerged as a critical and important problem for police, correctional, and medical care workers. The scope and magnitude of the problem clearly reveals that the subject matter is worthy of further consideration. Although the frequency of these deaths is very low, the criticality of its occurrence requires attention to the subject matter. The purpose of *Sudden Deaths in Custody* is to provide current information that addresses the issue from a number of perspectives. It is our purpose to assemble, under one title, current research that addresses the varying facets that underscore the nature of sudden in-custody deaths. The intent is to provide information that can further educate and assist those officers, administrators, investigators, trainers, and medical personnel who must interact, intervene, and make decisions about how to prevent sudden in-custody deaths.

*Sudden Deaths in Custody* specifically addresses sudden in-custody deaths that occur after a violent confrontation. Such incidents may occur after police or correction officers' intervention, but also include incidents that may occur in a mental health facility or emergency medical field setting. The deaths described in this volume all involve sudden death within minutes or hours of contact preceded by one or more of the following: violent confrontation with police or corrections personnel, forcible control measures, and behavior influenced by a chemical substance, or mental impairment. Incidents involving custodial suicides, homicides, accidents, fatal pursuits, or police shootings are excluded.

The contents of *Sudden Deaths in Custody* include an assessment of the medical considerations involved in these cases; how the stress of the encounter plays a role on the physiological responses of the subject; the influence of chemical substances on the behaviors of the violent person and their role in contributing to the death of the person; and an explanation of the role of excited delirium. Additionally, the book addresses the use of force by neck holds, restraints, aerosols, tasers, and other measures. Specific case examples are provided, which illustrate the nature and problems associated with these deaths, along with the issues involved in performing a custodial death investigation.

A description of the civil liability issues that emerge from custodial deaths is provided by examining case decisions surrounding them. Finally, administrative issues are addressed. These include risk management strategies, policy and procedure concerns, training issues, subject monitoring issues, transportation concerns, officer incident reporting, and investigating an incident from the agency perspective.

The contributors to *Sudden Deaths in Custody* include three forensic pathologists, six medical physicians, and one PhD. All of the contributing authors are experts in their fields, having researched and published information on this important subject.

*Darrell L. Ross,* PhD
*Theodore C. Chan,* MD

# Contents

# Contributors

THEODORE C. CHAN, MD • Professor of Clinical Medicine and Medical
Director Department of Emergency Medicine, University of California,
San Diego, CA

RICHARD F. CLARK, MD • Professor of Clinical Medicine, Division of
Toxicology, Department of Emergency Medicine, University of
California, San Diego, CA

VINCENT DI MAIO, MD • Chief Medical Examiner, Bexar County, San Antonio
and Professor, Department of Pathology, University of Texas Health
Science Center, San Antonio, TX

ELIZABETH A. LAPOSATA, MD • Department of Pathology and Laboratory
Medicine, Brown University School of Medicine, Providence, RI;
President, Forensic Pathology & Legal Medicine Inc.; Former Chief
Medical Examiner, State of Rhode Island, Providence, RI

TOM NEUMAN, MD • Professor of Clinical Medicine, Department of Emergency
Medicine, University of California, San Diego, CA

DARRELL L. ROSS, PhD • Associate Professor, Department of Criminal Justice,
East Carolina University, Greenville, NC

AARON B. SCHNEIR, MD • Assistant Clinical Professor of Medicine, Division
of Toxicology, Department of Emergency Medicine, University of
California, San Diego, CA

CHRISTIAN SLOANE, MD • Assistant Clinical Professor of Medicine, Department
of Emergency Medicine, University of California, San Diego, CA

GARY M. VILKE, MD • Professor of Clinical Medicine, Department of
Emergency Medicine, University of California, San Diego, CA

CHARLES V. WETLI, MD • Chief Medical Examiner, Suffolk County
and Professor, Department of Pathology, State University of New York
Stony Brook, Stony Brook, NY

# Chapter 1

# The Nature of Sudden In-Custody Deaths

*Darrell L. Ross*

## INTRODUCTION

The sudden death of an arrestee, a detainee in police/detention custody, or an individual confined in a mental health facility, after a violent encounter, is an unexpected event that can create a significant impact on the criminal justice system, the community at large, and the medical community. For a number of years, police, correction, and psychiatric entities have undergone sharp public, medical, and legal scrutiny regarding the type and degree of force that was used, as well as the type of restraints that were applied in subduing the resisting person. In a significant percentage of incidents the resisting person exhibits bizarre behavior, combative and violent resistance, requiring multiple personnel to respond and use higher levels of physical force, and varying types of force methods and restraint equipment. The resisting person's behavior is often related to chemical impairment, symptoms of mental impairment, or both. After restraint has been accomplished, responding personnel notice that the once combative person has become tranquil and unresponsive, requiring medical intervention. Efforts to revive the person by the responding personnel or emergency medical personnel were unsuccessful, whereupon it is determined that the individual is dead, all within a short time after the confrontation.

Normally, officers restrain a resisting person without sustaining serious medical problems as reasonable and legitimate force measures are used to control the violent person. In a few cases, however, the restrained person suddenly dies for

From: *Forensic Science and Medicine: Sudden Deaths in Custody*
Edited by: D. L. Ross and T. C. Chan © Humana Press Inc., Totowa, NJ

reasons not related directly to the physical aspects of the force methods applied or to restraint. Frequently, the autopsy findings do not demonstrate anatomic or toxicological results sufficient to explain the death. This does not, however, bring finality to the case, as these incidents most assuredly will culminate in a wrongful death civil action against the responding personnel and their agency.

The following case example depicts an illustration of such a sudden in-custody death scenario: police responded to a residence as a man in his 30s was physically threatening the home owner and destroying property. The individual was violent, delirious, and verbally uncooperative, appeared to be under the influence of a chemical substance, and charged the four responding officers. The police responded with physical force control measures and forced the man to the ground, handcuffed his hands behind his back, and restrained his ankles with a hobble restraint device (independent of the handcuffs) as he began to kick the officers. Within a matter of minutes, an officer noticed that the arrestee had calmed down, began to loose color in his face, and became unresponsive. The officers began resuscitation efforts and summoned paramedics. When the paramedics arrived, the individual was without vital signs. Paramedics began resuscitation efforts and transported him to the hospital, but he died en-route.

An autopsy conducted by the pathologist revealed numerous superficial contusions and abrasions, consistent with a struggle and fresh injection sites on both arms. The man had a lengthy history of prior cocaine and methamphetamine use. Toxicology analysis indicated blood levels of cocaine at 0.57 mg/L and benzoylecoginine at 3.8 mg/L. The cause of death was determined to be cocaine intoxication.

When a person suddenly dies in police custody after a violent restraint incident, concerns are created beyond the immediate interests of the law enforcement officials. Even when officers take proper measures to use "objective reasonable" force methods to control and restrain the person, he or she can still die. Death may be the result of respiratory or cardiac failure associated with heart and lung disease, heart conditions directly related to chemical abuse, abuse of recreational drugs, other internal organ deficiencies, mental impairment condition, or asphyxia. In many cases, however, the specific cause of death is not identified with medical certainty.

Regardless of the specific cause of death, the political fallout for the officers can be immense. An in-custody death can spark community unrest, ignite community protests, disturbances or riots, and intensify polarization between the police and the community. After one in-custody death in a midwest community, the family of the deceased filed a wrongful death lawsuit against the governmental entity, staged several protests, and purchased two billboards in the city announcing in bold letters: **"The Police Killed Our Father."** The sign was finally removed after 3 years when the officers prevailed in a federal civil lawsuit.

## THE PROBLEM

The central problem in a sudden restraint death is identifying the exact cause of death. Determining the manner and cause of death can be problematic as there are generally a myriad of factors that are involved in the incident. Although a sudden in-custody death can comprise innumerable factors, some of the more common features may include behavior and condition of the decedent, type of force and force equipment employed by responding officers, methods of restraint used by responding officers, methods employed for monitoring the person after restraint, thoroughness of the investigation after the incident, medical or psychological issues involved, thoroughness of an autopsy, influence of chemicals that the decedent may have consumed and toxicology findings, and determination of the manner and cause of death by the pathologist. These factors, as well as others, can present potential problems for responding personnel, their agency, death investigators, and pathologists, as they will more than likely encounter criminal or civil allegations. Clearly, the complexities of these cases require attention from the various personnel and entities that may become involved in the incident. There are three key areas that impact the nature of a sudden in-custody restraint death. Each is briefly described below.

### Use of Force

Sudden custodial restraint deaths have occurred during a confrontation between an individual and the police in varying arrest situations and in correctional and mental health facilities. One of the important components that emerge from a sudden in-custody death revolves around the control methods, force equipment, and the types of restraint employed by responding personnel to control the resisting person. Police and detention officers have been given the legitimate authority to use force to effect an arrest, to overcome unlawful resistance, in self-defense, to prevent a crime, to protect a third party, to protect the person from harming him or herself, and for medical intervention purposes. Medical care workers also have a legitimate need and interest in using physical control methods and equipment to control and restrain a combative patient for medical intervention and safety purposes.

Police and correction officers confront a wide variety of situations in the course of performing their duties. They can encounter situations that can range from a minor concern to a more serious lethal force incident. With some frequency, they also interact with individuals who exhibit various bizarre behaviors that may result from the influence of a chemical substance or a mental impairment. When dealing with these types of individuals the probability that an officer will have to use an elevated level of physical force increases *(1,2)*.

The problem is more than academic in that the police and correction officers encounter the mentally impaired or those under the influence of a chemical with some frequency. In a content analysis of 43 police use-of-force studies from 1968 to 2003, Ross reported that 65% of the studies revealed a significant percentage of the resisting individuals were either under the influence of a chemical substance or mentally impaired in situations where officers were required to use physical force measures or force equipment *(3)*. The officer also encountered multiple types of resistance, including verbal threats, defensive resistance, active aggression, and lethal force assaults.

Statistics on the annual number of sudden in-custody restraint deaths do not exist. In a significant percentage of use-of-force incidents, the police or correction officers physically control and restrain the violent person without the person sustaining a serious medical injury or death. Over the years, less lethal force technology has improved officers use-of-force decision making and response by allowing officers to choose various force options that provide for effective control and at the same time reduce the likelihood that the person or officer will incur an injury. Besides having access to physical force techniques and firearms, many officers have at their disposal such options as varying types of aerosols, impact weapons, tasers, stun guns, and restraint equipment.

In a significant percentage of incidents where officers employ these less lethal force options, the resisting person is controlled and restrained without sustaining a serious injury or death. The Ross analysis on use-of-force studies revealed that resisting persons sustained a serious injury in about 10% of incidents when less lethal force was employed *(3)*. Injury, however, does not necessarily equate with the use of excessive force by the officer. Three of the most comprehensive studies on police use of force conducted twice by the US Department of Justice (DOJ) in 1997 and 2001 *(4,5)* and in a similar study conducted by the International Association of Chiefs of Police (IACP) *(6)* in 2001, demonstrated that the police used excessive force in less than 1% of the use-of-force incidents.

The DOJ analyzed more than 44 million police and citizen contacts in both study periods. The DOJ found that in 1% of the contacts, the police used or threatened to use force measures. The findings showed that officers used handcuffs and physical force techniques in a majority of the force incidents. With less frequency, officers used aerosols, electrical devices, impact weapons, and firearms. The resisting citizen reported sustaining any injury in about 15% of the incidents and alcohol and the use of other drugs were influential in about 30% of the contacts.

The IACP study examined more than 45 million police calls for service, which included 177,000 use-of-force incidents and 8000 use-of-force citizen complaints over a 10-year period from 1991 to 2000. The police used force methods in 3.61 for every 10,000 calls for service. The prevalence of the use of excessive force was calculated at a rate of less than 1% in these incidents. The study showed that officers used physical force techniques and restraints, followed by the use of aerosols, electronic devices, and impact weapons, when confrontations required the use of force. Intoxication of the citizen influenced the types of resistance the officer encountered and the need to use force.

Overall, these studies show that police use of force is rare and that the use of excessive force is even more rare. The studies also show that citizens rarely incur a serious injury from the use of force, indicating that officers routinely use these same techniques and equipment safely. In rare cases, however, the resisting person suddenly dies *(7)*. What contributed to the death becomes the pivotal nature of the problem and a main question, among many, that will be vigorously debated. Moreover, individuals with the same behaviors and abuse of recreational drug who are not in police or detention custody, also die at their place of residence, in an ambulance, or in the hospital.

Balancing the need to use force and the amount of force required to affect an arrest or to restrain a combative individual requires officers to make sound and justifiable decisions. Police and correction officers are expected to use reasonable intervention techniques and force measures when dealing with impaired persons. At the same time, however, they must be concerned about their own safety, the safety of the person, and others. This situation can be problematic and places the officer in a precarious situation, one in which mistakes of judgment or tactics can result in negative consequences.

When officers use force and restraint measures in response to the violent resistance of a person, which have been used in numerous previous similar encounters without problem, and that person suddenly dies, they and their agency will likely be bombarded with such probing questions as those that follow here:

1. What type of force techniques did the officers use?
2. What type of restraint equipment did the officers use?
3. Were alternative restraint or force techniques available?
4. Did the restraining officers contribute to the individual's death?
5. What type of position was the person forced to assume? And for how long?
6. Did the officers conduct any medical/psychological assessment of the person?
7. Did the officers provide or delay providing emergency medical care for the person?
8. What was the manner of monitoring the person?
9. What was the manner of police transport of the person and to what location was the person transported?

These, and a multitude of other questions, will specifically be directed at the responding officers and their agency's supervisory personnel. A wrongful death lawsuit will most assuredly be filed, alleging that the officers were the proximate cause of the individual's death, used excessive force, and were also willful, wanton, and deliberately indifferent to the medical needs of the deceased.

## Medico-Legal Investigation

The second potential area that emerges from a sudden in-custody restraint death is determining the manner and cause of death. An integral element of forensic pathology is the correlation between the circumstances of death and the pathological and toxicological findings of the postmortem examination. A sudden custodial restraint death frequently demonstrates less pathological evidence than may be found in other death cases. With less anatomic findings, historical, circumstantial, and scene investigation information becomes of paramount importance *(7–12)*.

Because the responding officers will be under the cloud of critical scrutiny, a thorough investigation by police and medical personnel is necessary and critical in order to determine what contributed to the sudden death. These two entities should work in concert in order to render the cause of the death. Police investigators should closely examine all scene evidence and force equipment employed by officers. Investigators should also interview all involved officers, responding emergency personnel, and any witnesses. Obtaining historical information about the decedent is also important.

The pathologist should use caution in rendering a cause and manner of death. The pathologist should examine the scene before conducting the autopsy in order to fully understand the circumstances of the sudden death. An array of factors can be associated with a sudden in-custody death, such as chemical levels and combinations of chemicals in the person's system, stress of the restraint situation, heart and pulmonary disease, other internal diseases/abnormalities, and acute exhaustive mania/neuroleptic malignant syndrome, to mention a few. Because these cases frequently generate allegations of abuse and police misconduct, careful examination of the condition of the body at the time of autopsy is important. A thorough external and internal examination of the body should be completed in more detail than what is normally performed. Specimens for toxicology tests and other tests should be performed based on the history and the nature of the circumstances. A complete synthesis of the circumstantial and forensic information should be considered prior to certifying the cause of death.

Classifying the manner of death in a sudden restraint death case can be most problematic for the pathologist. The pathologist must determine whether the evidence supports a natural death, homicide, accident, suicide, or is undeterminable. Any classification of the manner of death can pose potential problems in that any party that may be adversely impacted by the decision may challenge the classification. In many jurisdictions, a grand jury or a coroner's inquest may be convened to review the case.

Compounding the problem further, in many incidents, the estate of the decedent may hire an independent pathologist to perform an additional autopsy. It is not uncommon in these cases for the second pathologist to classify the death in a different manner than the initial pathologist. Such decisions can spark numerous accusations regarding the death, fanning the flame of a cover-up or conspiracy. In this situation, the net of suspiciousness and potential liability has widened to include the medical examiner's office, the officers, and agency. In any event, careful thought and due consideration of all the circumstantial, historical, and forensic evidence must be performed in order to justify the manner of death.

## Legal Issues

A third major problem facing responding officers and their agencies are the various legal issues that can emerge from the sudden in-custody death incident. This can generally involve two levels. First, responding officers, and perhaps their immediate supervisors, may be investigated for potential criminal charges. The local prosecutor or the state's attorney general's office may review the case to determine criminal culpability. Furthermore, the US Department of Justice may conduct a criminal or civil investigation into the incident. Although criminal investigations are not common in these cases, officers and administrators should check their respective states to be aware of the potential investigation or charges that might result from such an incident.

Second, what is more likely to result from these cases is the filing of a Section 1983 civil lawsuit against the responding officers and their administrators in federal civil court. The wrongful death lawsuit will be filed against the officers on claims of excessive force, failing to recognize signs and symptoms of mental impairment or substance abuse influence, and failing to render or summon timely medical care for the decedent. Administrators of the officers will also be named in the lawsuit. Claims of failure to train, supervise, direct, and discipline the officers are commonly lodged.

These claims will be framed within the context that the officers and administrators violated the constitutional rights of the decedent and that the estate should be compensated for the loss. Although not all allegations lodged may withstand judicial scrutiny, officers and their administrators should be prepared to defend each of them. Defending these cases can be problematic, particularly if the investigation has been less than thorough, officers' reports are incomplete, pathological findings suggest the officers may have contributed to the death, or there are differing theories between medical personnel on the manner or cause of death. With the innumerable complexities of these cases, many have subsequently been settled out of court.

## SUMMARY

Although statistically rare in occurrence, owing to the shear number of police and citizen contacts that occur annually, a sudden in-custody death should be expected. Police and correctional officers frequently respond to and detain a segment of the population that manifests a mental impairment, a history of medical deficiencies, and a history of substance abuse that may increase their susceptibility to a sudden death. Each case contains enumerable variables and case-specific facts that must be examined from varying perspectives, including the police/correctional response, the medical explanations as to the actual cause of death, and potential legal issues that may emerge. This triad of factorial perspectives comprises the varying facets surrounding sudden custodial deaths and represent complex issues that are not always easily answered. In the chapters that follow, current research from these three areas is presented in order to increase the knowledge about the nature of an in-custody sudden death.

## REFERENCES

1. National Institute of Justice. Use of force by police: Overview of national and local data. US Department of Justice, Office of Justice Programs, Washington, DC, 1999.
2. Geller WA, Toch H. And justice for all: understanding and controlling police abuse of force. Police Executive Research Forum, Washington, DC, 1995.
3. Ross DL. A content analysis of the emerging trends in the use of non-lethal force research in policing. Law Enforcement Executive Forum 2005;5: 121–148.
4. Bureau of Justice Statistics. Police use of force: collection of national data. US Department of Justice, Office of Justice Programs, Washington, DC, 1997.
5. Bureau of Justice Statistics. Contacts between police and the public: findings from the 1999 national survey. US Department of Justice, Officer of Justice Programs, Washington, DC, 2001.
6. International Association of Chiefs of Police. Police use of force in America. International Association of Chiefs of Police, Alexandria, VA, 2001.
7. Di Maio D J, Di Maio VJ. Forensic Pathology. Elsevier, New York, NY, 2004.
8. Luke JL, Reay DT. The perils of investigating and certifying deaths in police custody. Am J Forensic MedPathol 1992;13:98–100.
9. Copeland AR. Deaths in custody revisited. Am J Forensic Med Pathol 1984;5:121–124.
10. Segest E. Police custody: deaths and medical attention. J Forensic Sci 1987;32:1694–1703.
11. Lifscgultz BD, Donoghue ER. Deaths in custody. J Forensic Sci 1992;39:45–71.
12. Eckert WG. Medicolegal investigation of problems involving criminals and criminal activity. Am J Med Pathol 1983;4:279–286.

# Chapter 2

# Medical Overview of Sudden In-Custody Deaths

*Theodore C. Chan*

Because of the large number of individuals who are in the custody of law enforcement at any one time, deaths of individuals can occur and should be expected. Estimates regarding the exact numbers of custody deaths vary, but roughly occur at a rate of 0.1 per 100,000 of the total population of citizens in a given community *(1)*. When these deaths are studied, well over half that occur in custody are attributable to natural causes *(2–5)*. These natural causes are primarily from heart disease, other atherosclerotic diseases, seizure disorders, and alcohol and drug abuse. A large proportion of the remaining deaths in custody are the result of suicide or homicidal and unintentional lethal acts of violence *(2)*. In many of these cases, the victim is simply found dead in the jail cell and a clear cause of death can be determined at the scene or on autopsy.

The sudden, unexpected death of an individual in custody during or immediately following combative confrontation with law enforcement personnel represents an entirely different matter. In general terms, *sudden death* has been defined and applied to the unexpected cardiac deaths of individuals who were in a stable medical condition less than 24 hours previously with no evidence of a noncardiac cause *(6)*. Although sudden in-custody deaths are similar in presentation, the cause of death is often unclear. In many cases, these individual are of a younger age and may not have a significant past history of prior illness or an underlying medical condition when compared with individuals who die of

From: *Forensic Science and Medicine: Sudden Deaths in Custody*
Edited by: D. L. Ross and T. C. Chan © Humana Press Inc., Totowa, NJ

natural causes *(2)*. These sudden, unexpected deaths often occur during arrest or soon after confrontation with law enforcement and early on in the course of the individual's custody *(1)*.

These types of sudden in-custody deaths share a number of similarities and patterns that have been termed the *in-custody death syndrome*. First, individuals are often in a state of combative agitation and delirium, which precipitates the response of law enforcement. This state can occur as a result of stimulant and other recreational drug abuse, mental illness, or other unknown causes. Second, these individuals are involved in a violent confrontation with law enforcement in which various force methods, restraint, and so-called "less lethal" technologies are used in an attempt to subdue these individuals. Third, the death is commonly described as an acute event in which the individual suddenly becomes "quiet," "calm," and unresponsive. At that time, the individual is noted to be apneic (not breathing), pulseless, and in a state of cardiopulmonary arrest, for which resuscitation efforts are ultimately futile.

Fourth, on autopsy, there is often no clear cause on pathological examination of the body to explain the sudden, precipitous death that occurred. Medical examiners are left to theorize about the potential contributors to the cause of death, including the individual's underlying medical condition (i.e., evidence of cardiac or pulmonary disease such as cardiomegaly), the acute state of the individual (i.e., acute psychosis or drug-induced state), and law enforcement use of force and restraint methods (i.e., neck restraint, less lethal weapons used). As a result of the complicated and less-than-absolute determination of cause of death, controversy can arise in which law enforcement and excessive-use-of-force methods are ultimately blamed for the demise of the individual.

Although these cases are of obvious importance to law enforcement, the sudden in-custody death syndrome is also of great interest to the medical community, not just from an academic standpoint, but also from a practical nature in terms of preventing these deaths and recognizing and caring for individuals at risk. Paramount to the evaluation of this syndrome is a number of key, critical questions that this text examines. First, what is our medical understanding and knowledge regarding the pathophysiology of sudden in-custody death syndrome and the state of current research on this topic? Second, are there identifiable risk factors such as drug use, acute psychosis, or other characteristics that can help identify individuals who are at risk? Third, what is the role of use-of-force methods, restraint, and less lethal technologies in these cases? Fourth, what is the epidemiology not only behind these sudden in-custody death cases, but also law enforcement use of force in general, and violent injury and use of emergency medical and psychiatric care for the similar, more numerous incidents that do not result in sudden death in our communities?

## THIS TEXT

The next few chapters address the myriad medical and physiology issues surrounding the sudden in-custody death syndrome. The authors for these chapters come from a wide spectrum of medical specialties, including emergency medicine, prehospital care, pulmonary and critical care medicine, forensic pathology, and toxicology. The authors are leading experts in their fields and are widely hailed as the premiere investigators of the specific issues relating to sudden in-custody death syndrome that they address. These chapters include a discussion of important medical definitions related to this syndrome, including the epidemiology of sudden in-custody deaths; the physiological and pathophysiological considerations when evaluating this phenomenon; the risk factors and common patterns seen in these cases, such as the role of illicit drugs; the role of use of force, restraint, and less lethal technologies in these cases; and a discussion of the importance of conducting a thorough and complete medical investigation into these cases.

The next three chapters deal specifically with the role of restraint and restraint methods in the sudden in-custody death syndrome. In the first chapter (Chapter 3), Dr. Gary Vilke, an emergency medicine physician with experience in prehospital care, discusses the long history, physiology, and impact of neck restraint holds. Although long used in martial arts, the neck hold came under increasing scrutiny as a potential cause of sudden in-custody deaths in the 1980s *(7)*. Dr. Vilke discusses the anatomy and physiology of the neck, and the impact of various law enforcement neck holds including the bar hold, carotid sleeper hold, and shoulder pin restraint and their potential to cause significant or lethal injury.

In Chapter 4, Dr. Tom Neuman, an emergency medicine physician and pulmonary/critical care medicine specialist, discusses the role of restraint body position, such as the prone and hobble position, and whether these positions have any adverse physiology effects, including the potential to cause asphyxiation or death by respiratory compromise. Dr. Neuman reviews the numerous case reports and reviews, as well physiological studies investigating the positional asphyxia theory as it applies to restraint *(8)*. In addition, Dr. Neuman discusses other factors potentially related to restraint body position, including the role of weight force, ventilatory capacity and oxygen consumption, and cardiac physiology.

In Chapter 5, Dr. Elizabeth Laposata, a forensic pathologist and the chief medical examiner for Rhode Island, discusses the role of restraint stress and sudden death. Physical restraint, in and of itself, produces numerous physiological changes, including activation of the acute stress response, that may play a role in precipitating or putting persons at risk for sudden death. Dr. Laposata reviews the neuroendocrine physiology associated with the acute stress response, including the "fight-or-flight" sympathetic "catecholaminergic rush" response, and its potential role in sudden cardiac death. Dr. Laposata also discusses the interaction between psychological and physiological stress response and how these factors may play a role in the sudden deaths of individuals who are restrained.

The next two medical chapters address the role of illicit drugs and the syndrome of excited delirium in association with these sudden in-custody deaths. These individuals come into contact with law enforcement as a result of their violent, combative, and agitated behavior. Most commonly, this excited delirium state is a result of illicit drug abuse, primarily cocaine, but also methamphetamine, LSD, PCP, and other stimulants. This state can occur with drug use, underlying psychiatric illness, or an acute psychotic break.

In Chapter 6, Dr. Aaron Schneir and Richard F. Clark, emergency medicine physicians and toxicologists, review the role of illicit drug use in sudden in-custody deaths *(1,9)*. Drs. Schneir and Clark discuss the epidemiology of drug use and sudden death, particularly focusing on the role of stimulant abuse, and review current animal and human studies investigating the effects of these drugs. They review the physiological effects including cardiac dysfunction, metabolic derangements such as metabolic acidosis and hyperkalemia (elevated potassium levels), hyperthermia, and seizures, all of which may play a role in precipitating sudden death. Finally, Drs. Schneir and Clark discuss forensic drug testing for these illicit drug, as well as treatment for those who have suffered a life-threatening ingestion of these agents.

In Chapter 7, Dr. Charles Wetli, a forensic pathologist and a chief medical examiner in New York, reviews the fascinating etiology and physiology of the syndrome described as *excited delirium* (also known as *agitated delirium* *[10]*). Dr. Wetli discusses the history of this syndrome, previously known by a variety of names including "Bell's mania," "lethal catatonia," "acute exhaustive mania," and "malignant catatonia" to name a few, and discusses the potential relationship between excited delirium and other syndromes such as neuroleptic malignant syndrome. He reviews the clinical presentation of excited delirium and the potential pathophysiological mechanism behind the syndrome, including its similarities and difference from cocaine and other stimulant drug overdoses. Finally, Dr. Wetli presents a number of different case examples to illustrate this syndrome and its important role in sudden in-custody death syndrome.

Chapter 8 discusses so-called use of "less lethal" force weapons and technologies and their potential association with sudden in-custody death cases. Dr. Christian Sloane, an emergency medicine physician, and Dr. Gary

Vilke review these technologies, particularly focusing on oleoresin capsicum aerosol "pepper spray" and the taser electronic shock weapon. They discuss reports of sudden in-custody deaths associated with the use of these technologies and the current scientific research assessing the safety of less lethal weapons in humans. In particular, the chapter focuses on the effect of oleoresin capsicum on respiratory physiology and taser shock on cardiac function in humans.

Chapter 9 discusses the important issue of forensic investigation by the medical examiner into cases of sudden in-custody deaths. The chapter is authored by Dr. Vincent Di Maio, a world-renowned forensic pathologist and medical examiner, who is the editor-in-chief of the *American Journal of Forensic Medicine and Pathology*. In this chapter, Dr. Di Maio reviews the key aspects of the medical examination and forensic investigation into sudden in-custody deaths, discussing the pearls and potential pitfalls of determining and certifying the cause of death in these cases.

Whereas the chapters just discussed focus on the medical issues associated with the sudden in-custody death syndrome, later chapters in this text address epidemiological case examples, administrative and policy relevancy, and liability issues that all touch on the myriad medical issues and questions surrounding these deaths.

Ultimately, sudden in-custody death syndrome continues to be of great interest to a wide variety of diverse medical and health disciplines and specialties. Emergency physicians and field medical personnel regularly care for victims (including the involved individual, law enforcement officers, and bystanders) resulting from these types of incidents. Forensic pathologists and medical examiners often must make difficult interpretations as to the cause of death and injury in these cases. Medical administrators of jails, prisons, and mental health care facilities are interested in understanding the risks and preventing the occurrence of the sudden death syndrome in their facilities. Psychiatrists and toxicologists have great interest in understanding the pathophysiology and medical care needs for individuals who present with acute psychosis as a result of underlying mental disability or illicit drug use. Similarly, epidemiologists will be interested in the occurrence of these types of incidents and their associated patterns in our communities. Finally, public health disciplines and violence prevention advocates will be interested in addressing the issues that can arise in these cases in terms of reducing risk of violence and fatalities caused by the individual as well as by the potential use of excessive force by law enforcement. We hope this text begins to shed greater scientific and medical light, knowledge, and understanding of these events for all who are interested.

## REFERENCES

1. Karch SB, Stephens BG. Drug abusers who die during arrest or in custody. J R Soc Med 1999;92:110.
2. Reay DT. Death in custody. Clinics Lab Med 1998;18(1):1.
3. Adelson L, Huntington RW III, Reay DT. A prisoner is dead: a survey of 91 sudden and unexpected deaths which occurred while the decdent was either in police custody or penal detention. Police 1968;13:49.
4. Copeland AR. Deaths in custody revisited. Am J Forensic Med Pathol 1984;5:121.
5. Frost RF, Hanzlick R. Deaths in custody. Am J Forensic Med Pathol 1988;9:207.
6. Priori SG, Aliot E, Blomstrom-Lundqvist C, et al. Task force on sudden cardiac death of the European society of cardiology. Eur Heart J 2001;22:1374.
7. Reay DT, Eisele JW. Death from law enforcement neck holds. Am J Forensic Med Pathol 1982;3:253.
8. Chan TC, Vilke GM, Neuman T. Reexamination of custody restraint positon and positional asphyxia. Am J Forensic Med Pathol 1998;19:201.
9. Stephens BG, Jentzen JM, Karch S, Wetli CV, Mash DC. National association of medical examiners position paper on the certification of cocaine-related deaths. Am J Forensic Med Pathol 2004;25:11.
10. Wetli CV. The history of excited delirium: characteristics, causes, and proposed mechanics for sudden death. In: Payne-James J, Byard R, Corey T, Henderson C. eds. Encyclopedia of Forensic and Legal Medicine, Elsevier, London, UK, in press 2005.

# Chapter 3

# Neck Holds

## Gary M. Vilke

The neck hold is a restraint technique in which a person is restrained by use of a hold that employs manipulation of the neck. Neck holds have been used extensively by law enforcement personnel for physically restraining and gaining control of violent subjects. Choke holds and carotid sleeper holds are types of neck holds that have been employed by law enforcement. Neck holds utilize the mechanism of temporarily disrupting the blood flow to the brain and rendering the subject unconscious. Additionally, neck holds have been used for decades in the sport of judo with tremendous safety. Occasionally, deaths have occurred during or just after the application of a neck hold and the etiology of the death is often attributed to the actual maneuver itself. In these cases, careful examination must be given to the type of hold, the application, surrounding circumstances, and the associated physical findings.

This chapter reviews the history and types of neck holds, safety, deaths, and clinical research associated with neck holds. The anatomy of the neck is defined to offer a better understanding of the effects these holds can potentially have on an individual. The different types of neck holds, including their applications, the potential risks, and complications, are discussed. Finally, there is a discussion about the management strategies for patients who are placed in neck holds and the potential need for medical assessment.

### ANATOMY OF THE NECK

The neck is a complex pathway of nerves, blood vessels, and airway, that when thought of in a most simplistic form, is essentially a relay system

From: *Forensic Science and Medicine: Sudden Deaths in Custody*
Edited by: D. L. Ross and T. C. Chan © Humana Press Inc., Totowa, NJ

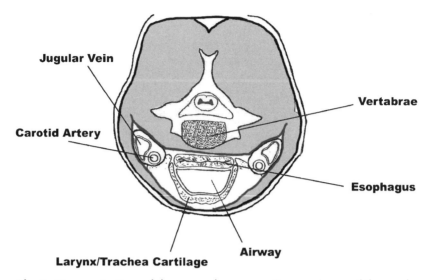

**Fig. 1.** Demonstration of the normal cross-section anatomy of the neck.

connecting the head and brain with the rest of the body. Neural transmissions go back and forth via the spinal cord, as well as a complex integrated system of nerve fibers. The brain is nourished by blood flow originating from the heart, transported to and from the brain through the neck. Regions of the neck regulate blood flow to the brain. This system includes specialized neuroendocrine and vascular tissue, such as the carotid bodies, which monitor blood pressure and blood oxygen and carbon dioxide levels, and adjusts blood flow parameters accordingly. The neck serves as a conduit for food and liquid of the gastrointestinal tract via the esophagus, and as a pathway to get oxygen into the lungs and carbon dioxide out of the body for the respiratory system. Disruption of any of these pathways or processes has associated physiological effects. Figure 1 shows the normal cross-section anatomy of the neck.

## Airway

The airway is essentially the breathing tube connecting the opening of the mouth with the lungs. It includes the pharynx, larynx, and trachea. Its function is to facilitate the passage of air from outside of the body into the lungs.

## Pharynx

The pharynx is the muscular posterior portion of the mouth that connects the oral cavity and nasal cavity to the larynx and esophagus. It is a passageway for food to the esophagus and for air to the larynx.

## Larynx

The larynx is a framework of cartilage that houses the vocal cords and is responsible for the production of vocal sounds. It serves as a passageway from the pharynx to the trachea. It is made of nine cartilages, which include the epiglottis, thyroid, cricoid, two cuneiforms, two corniculates, and two arytenoids that are bound together by ligaments and muscles. The prominence of thyroid cartilage of the larynx is often referred to as the Adam's apple.

## Trachea

The trachea, also known as the "windpipe," is the passageway for air from the larynx into the bronchial tree of the lungs. It is made of cartilage rings and lies just below the skin distal to the Adam's apple.

## Vasculature

The neck vessels are the conduit of blood to and from the brain, an organ that requires a robust source of oxygen.

## Carotid Arteries

The carotid arteries are the major sources of arterial blood flow to the brain. The common carotid artery on the left comes directly off of the aorta whereas on the right arises from the brachiocephalic artery that originates from the aorta. Both ascend to about the level of the Adam's apple and then divide into internal and external carotid arteries. The internal carotid arteries supply the cerebrum, forehead, nose, eyes, and middle ear. The external carotid arteries supply the face, scalp, and neck.

## Vertebral Arteries

The vertebral arteries transfer blood to the brain via a deeper route in the neck structures along the cervical spine vertebrae.

## Jugular Veins

The jugular veins are the major vessels draining the blood flow from the head.

## Musculoskeletal

The main bones of the neck include the cervical spine vertebrae and the hyoid bone.

## Hyoid Bone

The hyoid bone is a free-floating U-shaped bone in the anterior portion of the neck that sits below and supports the tongue. It is held in place by muscles and ligaments.

## Cervical Spine

The cervical spine is a series of seven vertebrae that are stacked on one another and house the spinal cord from the base of the skull to the thoracic spine. Between each boney vertebral body is an intervertebral disc.

## Neck Muscles

The musculature of the neck is a complex combination of small muscles attaching adjoining vertebrae and longer strap muscles that offer support and strength over the cervical spine as a whole.

## Spinal Cord

The spinal cord is the complex nervous structure housed within the cervical spine that runs from the brainstem to the lower portion of the spine. Its function is to transmit neurological impulses between the brain and the rest of the body.

## Other Related Structures

Several other important structures are housed within the neck region, including chemoreceptors, baroreceptors, and endocrine glands.

## Carotid Bodies

The carotid bodies are small, highly vascular tissues located in the wall of the carotid artery at the site of its bifurcation. The bodies contain chemoreceptors that monitor the levels of carbon dioxide and oxygen in the blood. If the blood oxygen level is noted to fall, the chemoreceptors send impulses to the cardiac and respiratory centers in the brain to stimulate heart rate and respiratory rate.

## Carotid Sinuses

The carotid sinuses are located near the carotid bodies and house baroreceptors that measure blood pressure coming to the brain. If blood pressure is low, the baroreceptors stop firing as they are no longer being stretched. Neural impulses are then sent to the brain via the glossopharyngeal nerve (cranial nerve IX) to triggering autonomic signals to stimulate the heart to beat faster and contract more forcefully, thus increasing cardiac output and improving blood flow to the brain.

## Thyroid Gland

The thyroid gland is a highly vascular endocrine gland located in the anterior neck just inferior to the Adam's apple portion of the thyroid cartilage of the larynx. Its function is to produce and secrete thyroid hormone.

## Parathyroid Glands

The parathyroid glands are four glands housed in the thyroid tissue of the neck that secrete parathyroid hormone, a regulator of blood calcium levels.

## Tongue

The tongue is a muscular structure that attaches from the floor of the mouth and has several functions, including taste, speech, and manipulation of food down to the pharynx.

## Esophagus

The esophagus is the muscular tube that transports food and liquid from the pharynx to the stomach. It is posteriorly located behind the airway and anterior to the cervical spine.

## HISTORY OF NECK HOLDS

### Use in Martial Arts

Shime-waza (choke hold) has been used in the sport of judo since its founding by Professor Jigoro Kano in Tokyo, Japan in 1882. According to a report by the Society for Scientific Study in Judo, shime-waza can induce a state of unconsciousness (Kodokan) from temporary hypoxia to the cerebral cortex *(1)*. The shime-waza hold results in victory when an opponent either indicates submission as a result of the technique or, having had the opportunity to submit, loses consciousness as a result of failing to do so. In both cases, it is accepted practice that the hold is maintained until the referee has announced the awarding of the point. The referees are typically trained to quickly detect loss of consciousness, and thus award the point and have the opponent release the hold *(2)*.

There are three forms of shime-waza: *okurieri-jime*, the neck being squeezed as a whole; *katajuji-jime*, the carotid arteries being compressed (similar to sleeper hold described later in the chapter); and *hadaka-jime*, compression over the trachea (similar to a bar hold). *Kesa gatame* is an additional judo position that utilizes lateral neck compression by pinning the subject's arms upward to immobilize and render an opponent unconscious.

Individuals placed in the katajuji-jime hold are often not uncomfortable. In fact, in more novice judo participants who do not submit, loss of consciousness frequently occurs. The more experienced participants recognize the position and its likely outcome and will more frequently yield and submit before they lose consciousness. This is in contrast to hadaka-jime, which becomes painful early because of the direct pressure over the anterior structures of the neck, including the airway cartilage, and usually results in submission by the person being choked well before loss of unconsciousness. The discomfort of okurieri-jime tends to fall in between these two techniques. Kesa gatame involves pinning the subject's arm up against the neck. The compression is over the lateral aspects of the neck and is typically not as painful as the hadaka-jime hold and can render a subject unconscious in short time.

Although there have been 19 reported judo fatalities, none were found to be caused by shime-waza *(3,4)*. Based on records from the International Judo Federation, World Class Championships, Olympics and Junior World Judo Championships reported in 1979, there were no reported deaths from the 2198 different techniques used to score, 97 (4.4%) of which involved the use of shime-waza *(5)*.

## Use in Law Enforcement

Neck holds have been used for decades by law enforcement agencies as a form of restraint in the continuum of the use-of-force progression. Typically, use of the neck hold is considered before moving on to more injurious force methods such as the baton and other weapons. The bar and the carotid sleeper holds are the two basic types of neck holds utilized. Law enforcement officers also utilize the shoulder pin restraint position, a third hold that has been taught over the past decade, as form of lateral neck restraint. Although law enforcement officers utilize several types of neck holds, they are often erroneously collectively called "choke holds," which is a term reserved for a specific type of hold that is elaborated on later in this chapter.

Similarly, confusion exists in terms of difference between strangulation and choking. Strangulation is defined as a form of asphyxia characterized by closure of the blood vessel or air passages of the neck as a result of external pressure on the neck *(6,7)*. Choking is a more vague term and refers to the violent act of strangulation, or aspiration of an object. "Choking out" or "choked out" is a term often used by law enforcement and medical caregivers when a subject has had a neck hold placed. It is not specific to any particular hold and does not

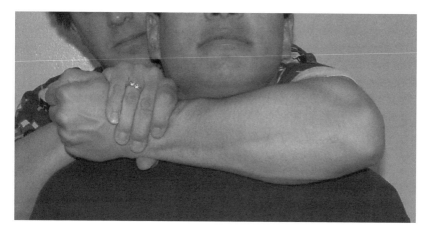

**Fig. 2.** Demonstration of the proper technique for placement of the bar hold.

necessarily mean that the subject was actually restrained to the point of loss of consciousness. This section reviews the types of neck holds and how they are placed.

## Mechanical Hold

Occasionally, a *mechanical restraint* will be placed on the neck of a subject utilizing a large flashlight, a baton, or other bar-like device, to compress the anterior portion of the neck. The hands of the restraining individual holding the bar device are placed around both sides of the subject's neck. The bar is pulled back, compressing the airway as well as the carotid arteries. The intent is to render the subject unconscious by compressing the carotid arteries and decreasing blood flow to the brain; or to gain control of the subject by submission owing to the pain and uncomfortable nature associated with the hold. As there is direct pressure from a firm object across the airway, injury to underlying structures, including the larynx, trachea, and hyoid bone is possible. Because of the risks associated with this neck hold, this technique has fallen out of favor and is not utilized as a primary neck hold by most law enforcement agencies.

## Bar Hold

The *bar hold*, also known as the *bar arm hold* or *choke hold*, is a restraint maneuver in which the forearm is placed straight across the front of the subject's neck while the restraining person is positioned behind the subject. The free hand grasps the wrist of the "bar" arm, and pulls backward putting pressure on the airway (Fig. 2). The intended mechanism for rendering the subject

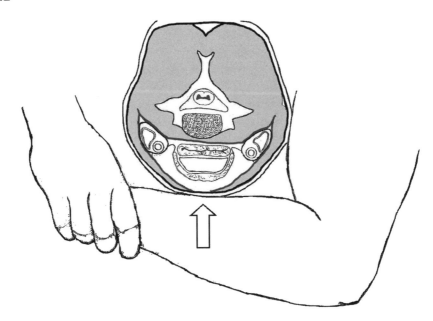

**Fig. 3.** A view of the neck in cross-section with the pressure placed on the anterior airway structures by the forearm when the bar hold is implemented. The notable features are the compression of the airway structures with more deformation, while the vascular structures are more spared in this hold.

unconscious is to occlude both carotid arteries, thus decreasing blood flow to the brain and inducing loss of consciousness. The risk of this hold is that too much pressure could cause airway injury, including laryngeal cartilage or hyoid bone fracture. Given the anatomic location of the carotid arteries along the lateral aspect of the subject's neck, the hold may not induce loss of consciousness from arterial compression (Fig. 3). This, in turn, may lead to greater force being applied and further potential for airway injury. Following loss of consciousness, the hold is then released. The unconscious state should last for approximately 30 seconds and if there are no associated anatomical injuries, recovery should occur in 10 to 20 seconds. Because of the associated risks of injuries and death to subjects, this hold has fallen out of favor for the safer carotid sleeper hold.

## Carotid Sleeper Hold

The *carotid sleeper hold*, also known as the *sleeper hold, lateral vascular neck restraint,* or the *carotid restraint,* is a maneuver in which the arm of the

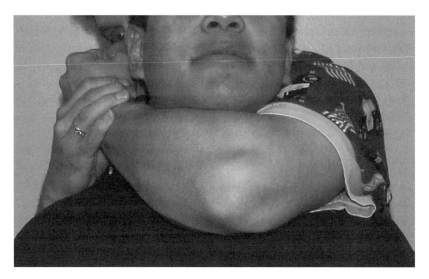

**Fig. 4.** Demonstration of the proper technique for placement of the carotid sleeper hold.

restraining person is held around the neck of the subject. The positioning is such that the crook, or anticubital fossa, of the elbow is over the anterior portion of the neck. The biceps region of the upper arm and the forearm are positioned to make a V-shape, with each region compressing the two sides of the neck. The free hand of the restraining person grasps the wrist of the restraining arm and pulls it back, thus creating a pinching effect (Fig. 4). The tightening of the arm compresses the sides of the neck, compressing the carotid arteries, diminishing cerebral blood flow and causing unconsciousness. Because there is a fulcrum effect of the elbow at the anterior portion of the neck, there is little pressure placed directly on the anterior airway, reducing the risk of collapse and injury (Fig. 5). When appropriately placed, the carotid sleeper hold will cause loss of consciousness within 10 to 20 seconds. At that point, the hold should be released and the unconscious period typically lasts up to 30 seconds or so after release. Theoretically, there should be no permanent sequelae after appropriate use of this hold.

## Shoulder Pin Restraint

The *shoulder pin restraint*, derived from kesa gatame, utilizes lateral neck compression to render the subject unconscious, but instead of wrapping the arm around both sides of the neck as in the carotid sleeper hold, one of the subject's

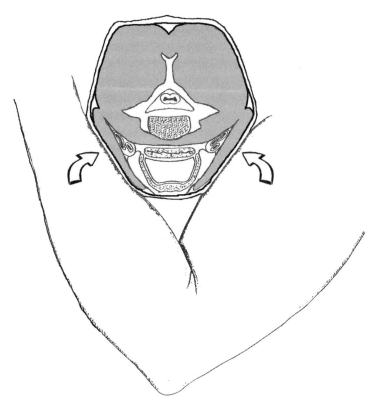

**Fig. 5.** A view of the neck in cross-section with force placed on it by a carotid sleeper hold. Note the compression on the carotid arteries by the forearm and upper arm, with sparing of pressure on the anterior airway structures by the crook of the arm when the carotid sleeper hold is properly implemented.

arms is pinned upward along his own neck (Fig. 6). The arm of the person placing the restraint is under the arm of the subject below the subject's shoulder girdle so that the subject's arm is forced to rise above his or her head. The wrist of the restraining arm is then placed on the opposite side of the subject's neck, just below the mandible. The elbow of the restraining arm is centered on the sternum. The nonrestraining hand grips the restraining hand and places pressure over the lateral neck of the subject. This hold, when properly placed, avoids pressure over the anterior airway structures, and with full compression, will render the victim unconscious in 10 to 20 seconds. As with the carotid restraint, the hold should be released when the subject loses consciousness, with the

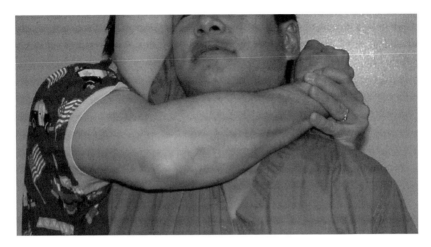

**Fig. 6.** Demonstration of the proper technique for placement of the shoulder pin restraint.

unconscious period typically lasting up to 30 seconds or so, with no permanent sequelae.

## REVIEW OF NECK HOLD-RELATED DEATHS

### Review of the Literature

Reay and Eisele were the first to report deaths from law enforcement neck holds describing cases of a 58-year-old man and a 35-year-old man who both had fractures of their thyroid cartilage on autopsy. The type of hold used in both cases was reported to be an attempted carotid sleeper hold that, because of the violent struggle, ended up becoming a bar hold *(8)*. Kornblum reviewed the case records of 33 deaths associated with choke holds. Many were associated with bar holds and several involved prolonged carotid restraint, from 1.5 to 3 minutes. He reports that 27 out of 33 individuals presented with abnormal behavior, 20 of which had confirmed toxicology screens that were positive for drugs or alcohol *(9)*.

Koiwai reported 14 fatalities in which autopsy findings determined that death was caused by the use of choke holds *(3)*. The holds utilized in these cases included mechanical holds utilizing a baton and a flashlight in two cases, bar holds in two cases, carotid sleeper holds in two cases, and unspecified neck holds in eight cases. All patients had evidence of injury to the neck, including bruises, ecchymosis, and hemorrhages on autopsy. Interestingly, five patients suffered fractures of neck bones or cartilage (cricoid cartilage [$n = 1$], hyoid bone [$n$ = 1], and thyroid cartilage [$n$ = 3]) and one of the intervertebral discs. These fractures occurred in subjects who died after either a mechanical hold or a bar hold. The other two cases occurred in a patient with a carotid sleeper hold and in a patient with an undifferentiated neck hold. Other deaths in this series were attributed to asphyxia, with prolonged holds after loss of consciousness. It should be noted that one of the patients had taken lysergic acid diethylamide (LSD), one had taken heroin, one had taken ethanol and cocaine, and three had taken phencyclidine (PCP). Several patients had heart abnormalities, including two with interstitial fibrosis, one with cardiomyopathy, and one with atherosclerotic hypertensive heart disease, although it is unclear if these abnormalities played any role in the actual deaths. Similar cardiac findings were also noted in a number of patients in Kornblum's report *(9)*.

## Controversial Use in Law Enforcement

Because of multiple reported deaths occurring in custody associated with neck holds, police and neck-hold techniques have come under scrutiny *(10)*. Kornblum, the acting medical examiner for Los Angeles County, wrote that a number of neck-hold deaths occurring in his county led to a series of lawsuits and court actions that jeopardized the continued use of neck holds. One of these suits led to the August 1981 ruling by the US Ninth District Court of Appeals that police officers could no longer use the choke hold unless "someone was threatened with serious bodily harm" *(11)*. In fact, a legislative proposal to eliminate the use of the bar hold and to classify the carotid sleeper hold as a lethal weapon, thus restricting use to life-threatening situations, was considered by the California State Legislature in 1983 but was not enacted *(12)*. Internal reviews with many agencies came to the determination that the bar hold placed individuals at risk for injury and death and this technique has been phased out of routine use by law enforcement. Many consider the use of bar or choke holds to be inherently dangerous because the design of these holds is to obstruct the subject's airway, or essentially to strangle the person into submission.

Kornblum also reported that when use of neck holds was restricted by the Los Angeles Police Department, a corresponding increase was seen in the use of fists and night sticks to subdue violent suspects. This led to an increase in injuries to persons being arrested as well as to police officers. Kornblum also reports that police officers preferred the control holds at the time, rather than utilizing the more brutal baton *(12)*.

In part because of these benefits, neck holds continue to be a common method of restraint by law enforcement agencies. Because concerns regarding the potential risk of the mechanical and bar holds exist, greater emphasis is now focused on the carotid sleeper hold. Use of this neck-hold technique is currently taught in many law enforcement agencies and is considered the hold of choice for safely gaining control of a subject. The technique is designed to render the subject unconscious in a brief period of time, while minimizing the risk of injury to the airway and to other structures of the neck.

## Anatomic Association

Deaths caused by neck holds are typically related to specific anatomic or physiological issues. These may be the result of underlying medical issues of the subject, or anatomic embarrassment caused by the actual hold, whether appropriately or inappropriately placed. Clearly, if a hold were maintained in position well after the subject has lost consciousness, continued obstruction of cerebral blood flow would lead to irreversible injury or death. It has been reported that neck pressure of 250 mmHg is necessary to occlude the carotid arteries, whereas the amount of pressure to collapse the airway is six times greater *(3)*.

## Airway Compromise

Bar holds directly place pressure on the anterior airway, which in turn may compress the airway, displace the tongue posteriorly and potentially occlude the upper pharyngeal region. Too much pressure can collapse the airway. This pressure across the airway is often evidenced on autopsy as fractures of the larynx, its appendages, or the hyoid bone *(13)*. A carotid sleeper hold is designed to better protect the airway, however, care must be used to maintain appropriate positioning, particularly in a struggling individual, as the hold could shift into more of a bar hold, and thus put the airway at risk for compromise.

## Vascular Injury

When a neck hold is used on patients with a significant medical history of atherosclerotic disease, they may be at risk for disruption of atherosclerotic material or plaque. This disruption of plaque can result in a stroke from blockage of blood flow in the carotid arteries. Such cases have occurred in the medical field with the use of carotid sinus massage. Carotid sinus massage involves placing pressure directly over the carotid artery at the level of the carotid sinus and massaging the area that has the effect of increasing neurological discharge to slow down the heart rate. Munro and colleagues reported seven episodes of the neurological symptoms consistent with brain ischemia in older patients with of the use of carotid sinus massage in 5000 patients. Munro's neurological findings included weakness in five patients and visual field defects in two. Of these cases, five spontaneously resolved, one had persistent residual weakness on the same side as a pre-existing stroke, and another had permanent visual field loss *(14)*. Richardson et al. had similar findings in 1000 patients over 50 years of age, with 9 patients reporting neurological complications possibly attributable to the carotid sinus massage. Of these nine patients, all but one spontaneously resolved and the ninth had persistent hand weakness *(15)*.

Fortunately, atherosclerotic disease in the carotid arteries is most commonly found in the elderly population, a group less likely to require the use of a neck hold. However, the disease could be present in younger individuals. In most cases, it would be impossible for the restraining individual to know if this was the case at the time the subject requires restraint as there are no physical attributes easily identifying a person at risk for stroke from compression of diseased carotid arteries.

## Carotid Sinus Stimulation

Carotid sinus stimulation has been postulated as a possible etiology for sudden death in subjects undergoing neck holds. As noted previously, pressure on the carotid sinus body causes a reflex vagal nerve discharge that can slow the heart rate. The belief is that marked compression of the carotid sinus can cause significant slowing of the heart (bradycardia) to the point of cardiac arrest and standstill *(12)*. This theory is based on the medical condition of carotid sinus syndrome *(16)* and reports that some individuals can have marked bradycardia induced by neck massage *(17)*. Kornblum also reports on this reflex action and that "in rare instances, pressure to this area can lead to reflex cardiac arrest and sudden death." However, he provides no reference for this statement *(12)*.

The determination of death as a result of carotid sinus reflex is essentially impossible to determine at autopsy, particularly when alternative explanations for the cause of sudden death, such as agitated delirium or acute drug intoxication, exist. In one reported case in which the cause of death was listed as cardiac arrest from carotid sinus reflex, the patient had no neck injuries found on autopsy. The individual had been restrained because of psychotic behavior and delirium tremens from alcohol withdrawal. A choke hold was placed and the subject died suddenly while the force was being applied. The medical examiner reported that the diagnosis "almost certainly represents" death from carotid sinus stimulation, but this finding was made as a diagnosis of exclusion as such a cause would essentially be impossible to confirm *(12)*.

Although reflex bradycardia has been noted in a number of studies, there have been no reported deaths or bradycardic events to the point of requiring cardiac resuscitation in any of these studies *(13,18,19)*. Moreover, the medical literature is replete with studies examining the use of carotid sinus massage as a diagnostic and therapeutic examination tool. In studies of thousands of uses on elderly patients, there were no complications of death or bradycardic events requiring treatment or resuscitation, even though this age group is traditionally more likely to have carotid sinus syndrome and more likely to be symptomatic from carotid sinus stimulation *(14,15)*. In fact, the diagnosis of carotid sinus syndrome, although well written about, is essentially unheard of in patients under the age of 50 years *(20–23)*.

Given that the sudden deaths associated with neck holds by law enforcement officers tend to be in younger subjects, the likelihood of carotid sinus stimulation syndrome is extremely unlikely. Additionally, in all of the clinical reports, reviews, and scientific studies of patients undergoing choke holds or carotid sinus massage, there have been no reported deaths or bradycardic events requiring treatment or resuscitation. Although an interesting theory, the carotid sinus stimulation cannot be blamed for these sudden deaths.

## Spinal Injury

Injury to the spinal column and spinal cord causing death from a neck hold is rare and typically associated with bar holds. In a case reported by Kiowai, a 34-year-old patient who died following a bar hold was found on autopsy to have intervertebral disc fractures between the third and fourth as well as fourth and fifth cervical vertebrae. There was noted abnormal mobility of the cervical spine and a transverse tear of the ligamentum flavum, as well as an acute spinal epidural hematoma formed at the level of the third through eighth cervical disc. Death was determined to be from asphyxia from neck compression in this case *(3)*. Kornblum reports two subjects who suffered cervical spine injuries during neck holds. The first was a 53-year-old man being detained by a citizen with an unknown type of choke hold, who on autopsy had third and fourth cervical vertebrae spinous process fractures and hemorrhage within the spinal canal that was pressing on the medulla oblongata. The second was a 34-year-old man who had a bar hold placed on him and was found to have hemorrhage in the anterior longitudinal ligament, an abnormal hypermobility of the vertebrae, an epidural hematoma and a contusion of the spinal cord on autopsy *(9)*.

In general, the large amount of force required to cause such injuries makes it extremely unlikely when a neck hold is placed properly. The spinal cord injuries reported appear to be those in which bar holds were employed, with the exception of the one case of a nontrained person utilizing a neck hold. Higher risk patients would be those with underlying cervical spine pathology such as ankylosing spondylitis or severe osteoporosis, who would be at higher risk for spinal injury with any neck manipulation.

## Review of the Literature: Neck-Hold Clinical Studies

Clinical studies on neck holds are predominantly performed on subjects with experience in judo or other related martial arts or on law enforcement officers. All of the studies have been in controlled scenarios with many not even going to the point of loss of consciousness from the hold. The focus of the studies tends to be noninvasive monitoring techniques in subjects who volunteer to be "choked out." Some of the techniques utilized included evaluating brain waves utilizing electroencephalographs (EEG) or using transcutaneous technology to measure blood flow.

## Electroencephalographic Studies

Very few clinical studies have been performed on the effects of performing neck holds on individuals. Rodriguez et al. assessed EEG and regional cerebral blood flow (rCBF) utilizing the xenon 133 inhalation technique in 10 judoka subjects undergoing katajuji-jime (carotid sleeper hold-equivalent) neck holds to the point of unconsciousness *(24)*. Baseline data of EEG and rCBF were obtained at rest. EEG monitoring was done during choking and for 10 minutes before and after the choking. rCBF was performed immediately after the recovery of physiological breathing. There were noted EEG changes (2–3 Hz δ waves in all cerebral regions but with an anterior predominance) that started about 10 seconds after initiation of choking that lasted for 5–6 seconds. These findings were similar to the EEG findings as compared with earlier studies, however, the clinical implications are unclear *(25,26)*. There was a slight decrease in rCBF in the measurement done after the choke hold was performed. These findings were not statistically significant, and they concluded that rates of recovery are variable and depend on the individual.

Rau and colleagues evaluated EEG findings in six healthy volunteers experienced in judo or ju-jitsu. EEG recordings were followed for 40 seconds, after which the volunteer was placed into a neck hold until he gave a sign to be released. None of the volunteers lost consciousness. EEG measurements continued for an additional 70 seconds. Average choking time was 8 seconds (SD = 1.8 seconds). They concluded that neck holds in judo might induce subclinical EEG perturbations *(27)*.

## Vascular Flow Studies

Reay and Halloway evaluated five law enforcement officers who had a carotid sleeper hold placed until the point of near loss of consciousness. Each subject would give a signal and the hold would be released. Facial cutaneous blood flow was measured using a laser Doppler system on the cheek. The cutaneous measurements are based on the laser detecting movement of red blood cells in the capillary beds. These researchers reported an 85% decrease in blood flow to the face and head. However, given the technique of measurement being used to determine capillary flow, it is impossible to determine if the measured difference was from a decreased inflow of blood to the head as reported, or a decrease in outflow from the head because venous outflow obstruction caused the measured decreased flow through the capillary beds. In all likelihood, the decrease in capillary flow was from a combination of decreased inflow and out-flow. Accordingly, it would be premature to state that the neck hold results in an 85% decreased blood flow to the head since blood flow to the head was never measured in isolation in this study *(28)*.

Raschka and colleagues utilized Doppler ultrasonography in subjects placed in a neck hold to demonstrate a significant reduction in end-diastolic flow in the mid-cerebral artery. Peak flow, mean flow, and end-diastolic flow were measured at baseline in nine judokas at rest and while juji-jime (a neck hold with use of hands to put pressure on the bilateral neck regions) was placed by a judo expert. The baseline peak flow was 85.3 cm per second, mean flow was 53.8 cm per second and end-diastolic flow was 37.9 cm per second. With the neck hold, the end-diastolic flow was reduced to 4.2 cm per second. None of the subjects lost consciousness during the study. The authors also measured pulse oximetry readings from a probe placed on the ear, reporting a decrease from a mean 97.9% baseline to 93.2% during the hold *(29)*. It is interesting to note that even though end-diastolic blood flow was reduced on Doppler, the oxygen saturation, an indi-rect measure of hypoxemia, did not decrease by any clinically significant amount. Of the nine subjects, only one had a saturation drop below 90%. The clinical sig-nificance of these findings still remains to be determined.

## *Hypophysio-Adrenocortical System Study*

Ogawa and colleagues evaluated the effects of neck holds on five judo subjects utilizing the okurieri-jime hold. Baseline and follow-up blood counts and urinalysis were checked in all subjects. Each subject was choked to the point of loss of consciousness, which took from 8 to 14 seconds and lasted from 10 to 20 seconds. All recovered without difficulty or complication. Transient decreases in pulse oximetry readings from an ear probe were noted with a base-line mean of 96% decreasing to 86% with the hold and returning back to base-line after removal of the neck hold. The authors also found increased total white blood cell counts as well as the level of 17-keto steroid in the urine, a hormone released by the adrenal cortex during stress. These are findings that would be expected as a result of the body's response to stress, thus the clinical applica-tions are minimal, but it did reflect that having a neck hold placed results in a physiological stress response *(30)*.

## EVALUATION OF THE "CHOKED OUT" PATIENT

Very little has been studied on the medical evaluation of the patient who has been the recipient of a neck hold. Much of the work has come from those who work with judo participants, but formal protocols or guidelines do not exist. For victims of strangulation, reviews have determined what imaging studies should be obtained for evaluation, but given the retrospective nature of these studies, there was no opportunity to assess for sensitivity or specificity *(31)*. An approach to evaluate the patient who has been "choked out" is described here.

### History-Taking

The clinical presentation, taken in context with the history, will drive what objective evaluation is indicated. Key elements that should be obtained regarding the neck restraint include what hold was utilized, if it was properly placed, how long it was in place, whether the subject lost consciousness, whether the hold was promptly removed after loss of consciousness, and whether there were any other forms of force implemented (i.e., chemical agents, taser, baton use). Other important clinical elements include how long the subject was unconscious, and whether the subject came back to an appropriate orientation upon awakening. Vomiting, shortness of breath, and hoarse voice are other symptoms of neck injury. Other traditional historical questions about past medical history, medications, drug or alcohol use, and allergies are also helpful if available from the subject.

### Physical Examination

The airway will need to be assessed for compromise, including normal phonation, ability to speak in full sentences, and lack of stridor. Examination should include assessment for tongue and facial swelling, swelling over the trachea, and speech and breathing patterns. Patients presenting with acute respiratory distress, including stridor, will need aggressive airway management. Mild hoarseness or sore throat will require careful vigilance for any deterioration in airway status that would require additional management. Although initial presentation with nonfocal findings is reassuring, close observation is important, particularly in patients with significant soft tissue trauma and bruising. Clearly, patients on anticoagulants are at increased risk for hematoma formation and airway compression and should be watched closely.

A careful neurological examination must be performed. Any abnormal findings would require additional objective evaluation. The examination should include cranial nerves, specific evaluation for Horner's syndrome (combination of lateralizing ptosis, myosis, and anhidrosis of the face indicating compromise of the cervical sympathetic nerves of the neck), motor examination, sensory examination, and cerebellar assessment. Finally, there should be a physical palpation of the neck. The cervical spine should have assessment for tenderness to palpation over the spinous processes. Additionally, the anterior components of the neck should be palpated with careful attention to the region over the carotid arteries and the anterior trachea. Range of motion should be assessed if there are no neurological findings and no tenderness to palpation over the spinous processes. The carotid arteries should be auscultated for bruits, and if none present, palpated for tenderness and thrills.

## Diagnostic Imaging

Imaging in the patient who had a carotid restraint placed is based on clinical findings. When determining which patients require imaging, the anatomic areas to consider include the airway; the spine, including the vertebrae and spinal cord; the esophagus; and the carotid arteries.

After appropriate steps have been taken to manage the patient's airway, imaging is directed at the patient's clinical presentation. All patients with stridor or change in speech require evaluation. Direct laryngoscopy or radiographic imaging including computed tomography (CT) scanning are two appropriate options. If there were evidence of aspiration or involvement of the bronchi, then bronchoscopy would be necessary. Careful clinical monitoring is appropriate for mild cases.

If there is suspicion for cervical spine injury, particularly if there is point tenderness over the spinous processes of the cervical spine, plain film radiograph is the standard imaging modality used. If there is clinical evidence of a cervical spine injury, then the patient will likely require additional imaging, including CT or magnetic resonance imaging (MRI). Although extremely unlikely in an appropriately placed hold, special consideration should be given to patients with increased risk, including elderly patients, patients with significant osteoporosis, and patients with underlying spinal pathology, such as ankylosing spondylitis.

Injury to the esophagus is very unlikely in carotid sleeper and bar holds. If there is injury to the esophagus, it will likely be in conjunction with injury to the airway as well. In a patient with significant injury, evaluation of the esophagus would be warranted, typically utilizing a swallow study or endoscopy.

The most challenging anatomic area to determine if evaluation is necessary lies with the carotid arteries. The injury that potentially can occur with blunt trauma is a carotid artery dissection (CAD). Dissection of the artery results from an intimal tear or primary hemorrhage of the vasa vasorum. Thrombus forms in the vessel and can lead to narrowing of the artery with reduced flow or the thrombus may break free and become an embolic source for distal branch occlusion causing stroke symptoms *(32)*. The patient with CAD will suffer cerebral infarction up to 82% of the time, and usually present within 7 days *(33)*. Alimi et al. reported that only 56% of patients present with clinical findings in the first 24 hours and 66% present within the first week *(34)*. However, symptoms of stroke have been delayed up to several weeks. In patients presenting with spontaneous CAD, the most common clinical findings include neck, jaw, or head pain; Horner's syndrome; and tinnitus in up to 96% of cases *(35)*.

Although CAD has not been reported in the literature in association with neck holds, evaluation of patients who had a neck hold placed on them often involves assessing for CAD. There are several imaging modalities used to diagnose CAD, including carotid ultrasound, CT, MRI/magnetic resonance angiography (MRI/MRA), and angiography. The imaging study of choice tends to be institution-dependent. Hughes et al. reported seven cases of blunt CAD in 3242 trauma patients over a 3-year period. These cases of blunt CAD were found coincidentally in six patients when MRI/MRA was being obtained to assess for soft tissue injury of the cervical spine and in the seventh when angiography was being performed to exclude a deep neck laceration *(36)*. Thus, deciding whom to evaluate with a radiographic study remains a common question. It is common for patients with abnormal, unexplained neurological findings after blunt trauma to undergo imaging. Additionally, imaging should be considered for patients with significant hyperextension or persistent lateral neck pain not consistent with paraspinous muscle strain solely after direct trauma.

The creation of a practice and treatment guideline has been made impossible by the infrequency of this diagnosis. Previous work has reported screening criteria to include neurological examination not consistent with brain CT scan, development of lateralizing neurological deficits (hemiparesis, transient ischemic attacks, cerebrovascular accidents, amaurosis fugax), Horner syndrome, signs of external cervical trauma, cervical bruits, basilar skull fracture and displaced mid-face or mandible fracture, massive epistaxis, severe flexion or extension cervical spine fracture, or neck hematoma *(37–39)*.

Owing to both the rarity of this diagnosis in blunt neck trauma patients, and the lack of a published case report implicating a neck hold as a cause for carotid dissection, it would clearly be acceptable practice to advocate reserving screening ultrasounds for patients with neurological deficits or findings of point tenderness over the carotid artery.

## FOLLOW-UP EVALUATION

Formal follow-up for these patients is not necessarily required; however, strict precautions should be given as to when they should be re-examined by a physician. These include any respiratory complaints, any new neurological findings, or difficulty swallowing.

## SUMMARY

Neck holds are a controversial subject. Clearly, their use in judo has a long history of safety, but the use of neck holds by law enforcement has been associated with cases of sudden death. Some of these cases have received significant media and public attention. The data clearly indicate that the bar hold technique can result in an increased risk of significant injury to individuals and, for this reason, should not be routinely used. The carotid sleeper hold, when utilized in younger subjects appropriately, has a relatively solid safety profile and is an appropriate form of restraint and use-of-force method in law enforcement's force continuum.

## ACKNOWLEDGMENT

The author would like to thank Morgan Carey for her assistance with the illustrations.

## REFERENCES

1. Tezuka M. Physiological studies of the Ochi (unconsciousness) resulting from shime-waza (strangle-hold) in judo. Bull Assoc Sci Stud Judo, Kodokan 1978;Report V:71–73.
2. Owens RG, Ghadaili EJ. Judo as a possible cause of anoxic brain damage. J Sports Med Phys Fitness 1991;31:627–628.
3. Koiwai EK. Deaths allegedly caused by the use of "choke holds" (shime-waza). J Forens Sci 1987;32:419–432.
4. Koiwai EK. Fatalities associate with judo. Physic and Sports Med 1981;9:61–66.
5. Barquin RC. Handbook of the International Judo Federation. 1979;29–39.
6. Iserson K. Strangulation: a review of ligature, manual and postural compression injuries. Annotated Emerg Med 1984;13:179–185.
7. Line WS Jr, Stanlery RB Jr, Choi JH. Strangulation: a full spectrum of blunt neck trauma. Ann Otol Rhino Laryningo 1985;94:542–546.
8. Reay DT, Eisele JW. Death from law enforcement neck holds. Am J Forens Med Path 1982;3:253–258.
9. Kornblum RN. Medical analysis of police choke holds and general neck trauma (part 2) Trauma 1986;28:13–64.

10. Reay DT, Mathers RL. Physiological effects resulting from use of neck holds. FBI Law Enforcement Bull 1983:52:12–15.
11. Lyons v. Los Angeles, 656 F.2d 417 (1981).
12. Kornblum RN. Medical analysis of police choke holds and general neck trauma (part 1) Trauma 1986;27:7–60.
13. Reay DT. Death in custody. Clin Lab Med 1998;18:1–22.
14. Munro NC, McIntosh S, Lawson J, et al. Incidence and complications after carotid sinus massage in older pastients with syncope. J Am Geriatric Soc 1994;42: 1248–1251.
15. Richardson DA, Bexton R, Shaw FE, et al. Complications of carotid sinus massage- a prospective series of older patients. Age Ageing 2000;29:413–417.
16. Cohen FL, Fruehan CT, King RB. Carotid sinus syndrome. J Neuroeurg 1976;45: 78–84.
17. Arnold RW, Dyer JA, Gould AB, et al. Sensitivity to vasovagal maneuvers in normal children and adults. Mayo Clin Proc 1991;66:797–804.
18. Arnold RW. The human heart rate response profiles to five vagal maneuvers. Yale J Biol Med 1999;72:237–244.
19. Berk WA, Shea MJ, Crevey BJ. Bradycardic responses to vagally mediated bedside maneuvers in healthy volunteers. Am J Med 1991;90:725–729.
20. Mallet M. Carotid sinus syndrome. Hosp Med 2003;64:92–95.
21. Kenny RA, Richardson DA. Carotid sinus syndrome and falls in older adults. Am J Geriatr Cardiol 2001;10:97–99.
22. Brignole M, Menozzi C. Carotid sinus syndrome: Diagnosis, natural history and treatment. Eur JCPE 1992;2:247–254.
23. Coplan NL, Schweitzer P. Carotid sinus hypersensitivity. Case report and review of the literature. Am J Med 1984;77:561–565.
24. Rodriguez G, Francione S, Gardella M, et al. Judo and choking: EEG and regional cerebral blood flow findings. J Sports Med Phys 1991;31:605–610.
25. Ikai M, Ishiko T, Ueda G. Physiological studies on "choking" in judo. Bull Assoc Sci Stud Judo, Kokokan 1958;Report 1:1–12.
26. Suzuki K. Medical studies on "choking" in judo, with special reference to electro-encephalographic investigation. Bull Assoc Sci Stud Judo, Kodokan 1958;Report 1:23–48.
27. Rau R, Raschka C, Brunner K, Banzer W. Spectral analysis of electroencephalography changes after choking in judo (juji-jime) Med Sci Sports Exerc 1998;30: 1356–1362.
28. Reay DT, Halloway GA Jr. Changes in carotid blood flow produced by neck compression. Am J Forens Med Path 1982;3:199–202.
29. Raschka C, Stock A, Brunner K, Witzel K. Changes of intracerebral blood flow during choking (shime-waza) in judo by transcranial Dopplersonography. Dtsch Z Sportmed 1996;47:393–398.
30. Ogawa S, Akutsu K, Sugimoto H, et al. Physiologic studies on "choking" in judo with reference to hypophysio-adrenocortical system. Bull Assoc Sci Stud Judo, Kodokan 1963;Report 2:107–114.

31. McClane GE, Strack GB, Hawley D. A review of 300 attempted strangulation case. part II: Clinical evaluation of the surviving victim.

32. Guyot LL, Kazmierczak CD, Diaz FG. Vascular injury in neurotrauma. 2001;23: 291–296.

33. Biousse V, D'Anglegan-Chatillon J, Touboul PJ, et al. Time course of symptoms in extracranial carotid artery dissections. Stroke 1995;26:235–239.

34. Alimi Y, Di Mauro P, Fiacre E, et al. Blunt injury to the internal carotid artery at the base of the skull: Six cases of venous graft restoration. J Vasc Surg 1996;24: 249–257.

35. Fisher CM. The headache and pain of spontaneous carotid artery dissection. Headache 1982;22:60–65.

36. Hughes KM, Collier B, Green KA, Kurek S. Traumatic carotid artery dissection: A significant incidental finding. Am Surgeon 2000;66:1023–1027.

37. Kerwin AJ, Bynoe RP, Murray J, et al. Liberalized screening for blunt carotid and vertebral artery injuries is justified. J Trauma 2001;51:308–314.

38. Biffl WL, Moore EE, Ryu RK, et al. The unrecognized epidemic of blunt carotid arterial injuries. Ann Surg 1996;223:513–525.

39. Fabian TC, Patton JH, Croce MA, et al. Blunt carotid injury: Importance of diagnosis and anticoagulant therapy. Ann Surg 1996;223:513–525.

# Chapter 4

# Positional and Restraint Asphyxia

*Tom Neuman*

## INTRODUCTION

The use of physical restraint to control violent, uncooperative, or combative individuals is to be expected in the law enforcement setting. Furthermore, the more violent, combative, or uncooperative an individual, the greater and greater degrees of force required to restrain such persons. When an individual dies under such circumstances, it becomes a legitimate question whether the restraint process or specific method itself had any causal relationship with the death or whether the death was predicated more upon the circumstances that led to restraint in the first place. Clearly, certain methods of restraint have been reported to be potentially harmful to individuals and as a result, certain "choke hold" maneuvers are no longer used by most police or law enforcement agencies because of the risk they apparently represent *(1,2)*.

Similarly the "hogtie," "hobble," or maximal restraint position has also come under scrutiny as a possible factor in the deaths of individuals being brought into custody *(3)*. In these positions, individuals are bound in the prone position with their arms handcuffed behind their backs and their knees flexed with their ankles bound together and then secured (with varying degrees of freedom) to the handcuffs *(see* Figs. 1 and 2). The literature includes multiple reports of deaths of individuals placed into these (or similar) positions, and the conclusion of some authors has been that the deaths were directly attributable to the restraint positioning *(4–6)*. The rationale for this conclusion was that the position impaired the ability of the individual to breathe and ventilate to such a degree that hypoxemia (low oxygen levels in the blood) secondary to

From: *Forensic Science and Medicine: Sudden Deaths in Custody*
Edited by: D. L. Ross and T. C. Chan © Humana Press Inc., Totowa, NJ

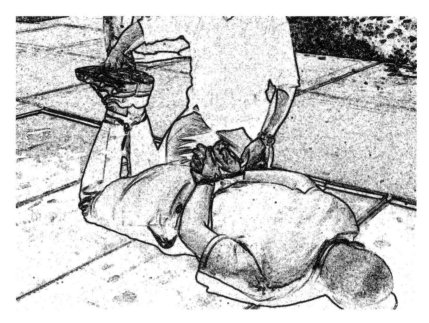

**Fig. 1.** Hobble prone restraint position. The position is similar to the hogtie position, but there is greater distance between the wrist and ankles when secured together allowing less flexion of the knees.

hypoventilatory failure occurred, and that the degree and duration of the hypoxemia was sufficient to cause death. With the understanding that this argument is predicated on certain pathophysiological processes taking place, it is worthwhile to review, albeit briefly, the normal physiology of the most important aspects of respiration.

## GAS EXCHANGE AND VENTILATION

Ultimately, the process of asphyxiation is the death of the individual and the associated failure of critical organ systems owing to lack of oxygen delivery. The delivery of appropriate amounts of oxygen to the tissues of the body is dependent on a variety of factors. For the purposes of this chapter, the most important factor is that oxygen actually gets into the blood (oxygen transport from the blood to tissues is assumed). Oxygenation of the blood is in turn dependent on two major processes. First and foremost is ventilation. Adequate amounts of gas must be delivered to the lung tissue or alveoli in order for proper oxygenation of the blood to occur (movement of gas also requires that the airway is patent). Assuming adequate ventilation takes place, then appropriate gas

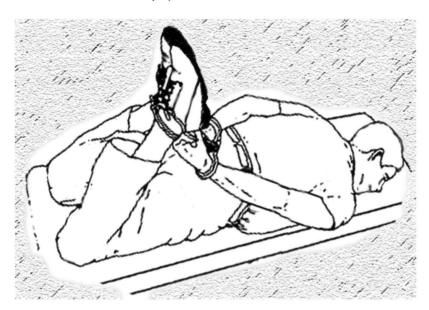

**Fig. 2.** Hogtie prone restraint position. The individual is bound in the prone position with arms handcuffed behind the back and knees flexed with ankles bound together and secured to the handcuffs.

exchange must also occur in order to assure oxygen delivery to the blood and subsequently to the tissues.

Ventilatory parameters can generally be measured by standard pulmonary function testing with spirometric functions being the most useful parameters to examine when looking at measures of gas movement. Measurement of gas exchange can be more difficult, however, the alveolar-arterial oxygen ($[A\text{-}a]O_2$) gradient is probably the most useful screening parameter to quantitate gas exchange. This number is calculated from the following equation:

$$(A\text{-}a)O_2 \text{ gradient} = (FIO_2 \times P_B - PaCO_2/RQ) - PaO_2$$

where $FIO_2$ is the fraction of inspired oxygen tension, $P_B$ is the barometric pressure, $PaCO_2$ is the partial pressure of carbon dioxide in the arterial blood, RQ is the respiratory quotient (respiratory exchange ratio) and $PaO_2$ is the partial pressure of oxygen in the arterial blood. A normal $(A\text{-}a)O_2$ gradient is less than 10–15 mmHg *(7)*.

A normal-sized individual in a resting state has a tidal volume of approximately 500 cc per breath. With a normal ventilatory rate of 12–16 at rest. This represents a baseline minute ventilation of approximately 6–8 L per minute. Vital capacity is defined as the amount of air an individual can take into his or

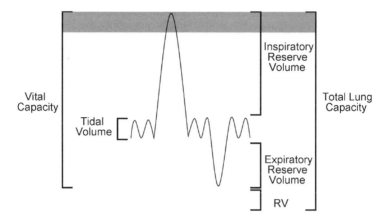

**Fig. 3.** Graph of lung volumes. Tidal volume is the volume of air in a normal breath in an adult (approximately 500 cc). Inspiratory reserve volume is the volume of air associated with maximal inspiration (excluding tidal volume). Expiratory reserve volume is the volume of air associated with maximal expiration (excluding tidal volume). The residual volume (RV) is the remaining air in the lungs after maximal expiration. Vital capacity is defined as the amount of air an individual can take into his or her lungs after a maximal inspiration (tidal volume plus inspiratory and expiratory reserve volumes). The 13% decrease in forced vital capacity with the hogtie restraint position is shown by the shaded region. The graph demonstrates the tremendous pulmonary reserve that minimize the impact of any respiratory decrement seen with the restraint position.

her lungs after a maximal inhalation. Figure 3 demonstrates various measures of lung volume. Forced expiratory volume in 1 second ($FEV_1$) is defined as the volume of air one can blow out in 1 second after a maximal inhalation and the forced vital capacity (FVC) is the volume of air one can blow out after a maximal inhalation. Finally, the $FEV_1$:FVC ratio is a parameter often examined as part of routine pulmonary function testing and in normals it is about 83% *(7)*. Pulmonary function testing also reveals that a person instructed to breathe as rapidly and deeply as possible for a period of about 30 seconds achieves a maximum voluntary ventilation (MVV) of about 160–180 L per minute.

A normal person has tremendous reserves in his or her ability to ventilate. At maximal workloads ($\dot{V}O_2max$), most individuals do not approach a level of ventilation that exceeds 70% of their MVV. Indeed, once an individual passes the age of 30 years, this percentage drops off even further because maximal oxygen consumption is dictated by cardiac output rather than ventilation *(8)*. Thus, it should be obvious that in order for a person to asphyxiate (from any cause) a dramatic reduction in the ability to ventilate must occur.

## HISTORY

Although a number of deaths have certainly occurred in individuals who have been placed in restraint positions, the actual physiological role of the restraint position in these deaths is unclear. There is no question that the entity of positional asphyxia exists. The term was apparently first used by Bell in a study *(9)* describing the deaths of 30 individuals in Broward County, Florida. No other significant risk factors for death were noted in this original description of positional asphyxia. The unifying feature of the vast majority of these deaths was that the individuals were discovered in positions that resulted in upper airway obstruction. These situations included hyperflexion of the head and neck or lying face down on a suffocating object. Alcohol intoxication (or other depressant drugs) was a major risk factor in these cases as well, and explained why these victims did not move from the position that caused the upper airway obstruction. In four cases, the torso was found to be hyperflexed accounting for a mechanical inability to breathe.

Another form of asphyxia has been termed *mechanical asphyxiation*. This has been associated with the use of a vest, jacket, or even posey restraints, and primarily has been described in the geriatric nursing home population. In this situation, asphyxiation occurs when these restraints accidentally wrap around the necks of the individuals and the result is simple strangulation *(10–13)*. In other cases, individuals became suspended from either a bed or a chair by their restraints with resulting chest constriction to the point of mechanical ventilatory impairment and death *(14,15)*. Thus, in its original form, the term *positional asphyxiation* described, in the vast majority of cases, either upper airway obstruction secondary to the position of the individual or simple strangulation owing to the position.

## CASE REPORTS

A number of case reports document the deaths of individuals who are restrained by law enforcement. However, these reports can only infer the role of the restraint in these deaths. Examining these reports reveals a pattern of deaths that is, without question, repetitive. In 1985, Wetli and Fishbain reported seven cases of deaths in cocaine users *(16)*. In their report, these researchers noted that five individuals were in police custody at the time and that four were placed in hogtie-like restraint positions. These authors suggested that the amounts of cocaine found in these victims did not support a simple diagnosis of cocaine overdose. They felt that the exact cause of death was unknown and speculated that the deaths might be the result of "autonomic reflexes, a toxic cardiac dysrhythmia, or 'restraint stress'."

Since this report, others have proposed that this position impairs normal ventilatory function and places such individuals at risk for death by asphyxiation. Based on this postulate, the term *positional asphyxia* has been used to describe these deaths, which appears to represent an entirely different syndrome than what was initially associated with the term in the past, as noted earlier. In 1992, Reay reported three deaths that occurred in individuals who were restrained and placed in the back of police cars *(6)*. All of the victims were violent, agitated, and uncooperative as a result of the use of various intoxicants or psychiatric illness. Assistance by multiple police officers was required in order to subdue these individuals and each one became unresponsive during transport. At autopsy, no clearly defined anatomic cause of death could be determined and it was concluded that these deaths were the result of the combined ventilatory effects of the semi-prone position and the confined space of the patrol cars.

Also in 1992, the San Diego Police Department, in conjunction with the County Medical Examiner's Office, formed a Custody Death Task Force to examine the issues surrounding in-custody deaths. This effort was spurred by seven in-custody deaths, three of which occurred in individuals placed in the hogtie restraint position. The task force conducted a survey of law enforcement agencies nationwide. Approximately 40% of these agencies reported experiencing in-custody deaths. The task force was able to confirm 94 cases of restraint-associated in-custody deaths during the previous decade, however, data collection was incomplete. Approximately 30% of the reporting agencies allowed the use of the hogtie position by officers to control violent individuals. The actual number of hogtie-associated deaths was not determined *(3)*.

In 1993, O'Halloran and Lewman reported 11 cases of sudden death occurring in subjects placed in the prone position. Nine of these individuals were in the hogtie restraint position. All of the subjects were combative, violent, and in an "excited delirious state" as a result of acute psychosis or drug ingestions (most commonly cocaine). Violent confrontation and struggle occurred in all cases. Two of these individuals were subjected to stun-gun shocks shortly before death. The authors asserted that the position "clearly impairs breathing in situations of high oxygen demand by inhibiting chest wall and diaphragmatic movement" *(4)*. In 1995, Stratton et al. were the first to report two individuals who died in the care of prehospital personnel and who had been placed in the prone restraint position for transport because of violent, agitated, and combative behaviors. Both were under the influence of drugs. The authors stated that the prone restraint position leads to "restriction of motion of the diaphragm and chest," and that such positioning "can lead to asphyxia" *(5)*. In 1996, Ross reviewed 22 cases of sudden death in the prone or hogtie position reported in the medical literature from 1988 to 1993. Of these deaths, 18 occurred in individuals in the hogtie restraint position, 2 were restrained prone on gurneys, and 2 were manually restrained in a prone position. All exhibited violent, combative behavior and fought or struggled with police. Drug use or alcohol intoxication was noted in 16 cases. Cocaine was noted in 12 subjects. Positional asphyxia was listed as the sole cause of death in 5 cases and as a contributing cause of death along with drug intoxication in another 6 cases. Ross concluded that placing a subject in a "confining position which restricts the natural respiratory process" can be fatal and that "based on the risk of sudden death the practice of hogtying and transporting subjects in a prone position should be discontinued" *(17)*.

## EXPERIMENTAL STUDIES

As should be apparent in all of the cases described here, the diagnosis of positional asphyxia is one of exclusion, as there were no experimental validation of these diagnoses other than prior literature stating that positional asphyxia occurred in these circumstances. The report that all of the above authors (except the first by Wetli) used as a reference to substantiate that the deaths were secondary to respiratory embarrassment was a study by Reay et al. published in 1986 examining the effects of the hogtie position. As this study was the single experimental reference used to supply a physiological rationale for the diagnosis of positional asphyxia in these cases, it is reasonable and probably critically important to carefully examine the methodology, the statistics, and the conclusions of that study in order to better understand the basis for the diagnosis of "positional asphyxia" secondary to the hogtie, hobble, or maximum restraint position.

Reay and his colleagues studied 10 healthy individuals who were placed in the hogtie restraint position or a sitting control position after a period of exercise on a stationary cross-country ski machine that raised the heart rate of the subjects to approximately 120 beats per minute. The authors noted a decline in peripheral oxygen saturation to 85–90% measured by pulse oximeter in these subjects during exercise. The authors then reported statistically significant physiological differences between the group in the hogtie position and the group in the sitting position after the period of exercise. Overall, the subjects in the restraint position had prolonged recovery times after exercise for both heart rate (approximately 35 seconds longer for the restraint group) and peripheral oxygen saturation (approximately 20 seconds longer for the restraint group). On the basis of these findings, Reay postulated, and all of the authors previously mentioned here accepted, the construct that deaths in individuals placed in the hogtie restraint position were the result of adverse respiratory effects from the body position. Reay further argued that the prone restraint position restricts chest and abdominal movement and therefore reduces ventilatory excursions, placing individuals at risk for hypoventilation hypoxemia and asphyxiation (18).

Before accepting these results, there are some significant methodological and conceptual issues that must be considered. Most importantly, this study is based on the presumption that exercise reduces peripheral oxygen saturation to 85–90% in healthy subjects. Unfortunately, this presumption is at odds with our current understanding of the effects of exercise on gas exchange. In contrast to Reay's observations, previous well-established work in exercise physiology demonstrates that arterial oxygenation improves rather than decreases with moderate exercise in healthy individuals (19,20). This occurs because pulmonary blood flow increases with exercise (i.e., cardiac output increases), and ventilation perfusion ratios throughout the differing lung zones improve, reducing the $(A-a)O_2$ gradient and also lowering $PaCO_2$ with still higher levels of exercise (19).

Reay's work is apparently predicated on his observation that oxygen saturation declines with exercise and this in turn was owing to the inappropriate selection of a transcutaneous pulse oximeter to measure oxygen saturation in his exercising subjects (21–23). Arterial blood gas analysis remains the preferred and more accurate method of measuring $PaO_2$. Indeed, it is well documented that potentially inaccurate results may be obtained from pulse oximetry when used on exercising subjects (21–23). Second, there appears to be another conceptual flaw in Reay's work. Looking at the data reported by Reay, his conclusion that the differences were statistically significant can only be duplicated if one uses a one-tailed $t$-test to analyze his results. Unfortunately, his work requires the use of a two-tailed $t$-test and if his analysis is repeated using the appropriate statistical methodology the results are no longer statistically significant. Third, even if hypoxemia actually occurred in his subjects following exercise, the hogtie position did not worsen that hypoxemia; it merely prolonged the recovery by 20 seconds (not statistically significant), which does not really support the concept that the hogtie position "causes" asphyxiation. Finally, although heart rate and pulse oximetry measurements were taken in these subjects, no direct measurements of ventilatory function were performed. Given the authors postulate that the hogtie position causes inadequate chest wall and diaphragmatic movements to the point of respiratory failure, it would seem crucial to measure parameters of ventilation. As this article is the sole scientific basis for all of the above-mentioned conclusions concerning the hogtie position, the claims that this position is inherently dangerous must be viewed with considerable skepticism.

Other more recent work more directly assesses the physiological impact of the hogtie position and gives considerably different results than the work of Reay *(24)*. A study by Chan and his colleagues in 1996 was the first attempt to critically evaluate the physiological consequences of the hogtie position. In this study, volunteers had baseline pulmonary function studies performed in the sitting prone and supine positions. Following this phase, the volunteers were then exercised to a mean heart rate of almost 170 on a bicycle ergometer and then placed either in a standard sitting position or in a hogtie position. Pulmonary function tests were repeated over a 15-minute period and blood gas determinations were made in triplicate from a sample of blood taken from the radial artery via a catheter that was inserted prior to the initiation of the study. The results of the spirometric studies revealed trivial changes in FVC, $FEV_1$, and $FEV_1/FVC$ ratios. These changes were approximately 7% in the prone and supine position and 13% in the hogtie position. The impact of the 13% decline in FVC is graphically displayed in Fig. 3. MVV decreased slightly more with declines of 10, 15, and 23% of predicted values.

Of more importance, however, was that arterial blood gas analyses revealed no change in arterial partial pressure of oxygen ($PaO_2$) and in arterial partial pressure of carbon dioxide ($PaCO_2$) between the two groups. The latter is particularly important, as it demonstrates no functional effect at all on ventilation from the combination of the hogtie position plus heavy exercise. It is also important to note that these findings persisted for the entire 15-minute period, during which subjects were in the hogtie position following heavy exercise. As would be expected, $(A-a)O_2$ gradient decreased with exercise and the $PaO_2$ increased when individuals' oxygen consumption exceeded the anerobic threshold. These finding are consistent with and expected based on prior work in exercise physiology *(19,20)*.

Schmidt also completed a similar study to that of Reay's and again found markedly different results *(25)*. In this study, 18 volunteers were monitored with baseline measurements and then were exercised on a stationary bicycle to a mean heart rate of 120 beats per minute. Heart rate and oxygen saturation were the parameters studied and no differences were noted in the mean heart rate or in oxygen saturation between the group in the sitting position and the group in the hogtie position. Following this, the subjects were further monitored after more vigorous exercise, which was intended to simulate pursuit and physical struggle. Again, no differences of heart rate or oxygen saturation were noted between the two groups.

Chan and his co-workers have also conducted a second study of the "hobble restraint position" *(26)*. This position is in many respects is the same as the "hogtie" position, but the knees of the subject are not as severely flexed as in the hogtie position. The hands continue to be restrained behind the individuals back and the legs are tethered to the wrists, with the knees only flexed to about 90° rather than a tauter position. In this second study, the effects of the hobble position combined with the inhalation of "pepper spray" were compared to the sitting position with and without pepper spray. Once again, no important physiological effects of either the spray, the position or the combination of the two were noted. The same minor changes in ventilatory parameters noted in their first study were again confirmed.

More recently, Parkes *(27)* attempted to duplicate Reay's 1988 study. Sixteen subjects were exercised on a bicycle ergometer to a mean heart rate of 120. At that point they were placed in either a seated, supine, or restraint position. No changes in oxygen saturation between the groups was noted, confirming the findings of Chan. Analysis of their data also reveals no significant difference in the heart rate recovery times between the seated and restraint position although they note a difference between the supine position and the restraint position. Unfortunately, an ANOVA was not performed to confirm the significance of these differences.

## POSITIONAL ASPHYXIA VERSUS RESTRAINT ASPHYXIA

Despite these carefully performed studies, authors have still ascribed the cause of death of individuals who have been maximally restrained to asphyxia. As it has now been shown that the hogtie position is physiologically of no consequence, it has now been opined *(28)* that the root cause of "asphyxia" in these cases is downward pressure on the back interfering with ventilatory mechanics rather than the previously indicted hogtie position. That is, asphyxiation occurs not as a result of position ("positional asphyxia"), but as a result of the actual restraint process ("restraint asphyxia").

In addition, it is further speculated that the weight of the individual (particularly if obese) while in a prone or restrained position is supposed to cause upward pressure on the diaphragm, interfering with its downward excursion, which in turn causes functionally important hypoventilation potentially causing "asphyxia." As with the previous hypothesis concerning the hogtie position, this construct needs to be examined very carefully in light of other clinical experiences and keeping in mind the paucity of experimental evidence that exists in this arena.

*ASPHYXIATION AND VENTILATORY REQUIREMENTS*

In order to examine the likelihood that an individual might succumb to asphyxiation from weight applied to the back during the struggle to restrain the subject, one must understand the process of asphyxiation. By and large, asphyxiation is the death of the organism secondary to the failure to deliver oxygen to critical tissues and the subsequent failure of critical organ systems. When oxygen delivery fails, either because of inadequate ventilation or inadequate gas exchange, the process is called asphyxiation. Because there are sizable oxygen stores in the body in the form of air in the lungs as well as oxygen in the blood, asphyxiation is a process that takes a considerable period of time in most circumstances. Thus, death does not occur immediately when breathing stops and the process of asphyxiation takes several minutes to occur even when breathing is completely arrested. Should small amounts of breathing continue the process takes even longer.

The critical question then becomes just how much ventilation is necessary in order for someone to survive. In the setting of thoracic surgery, when considering the likelihood that someone will survive a pulmonary resection for lung cancer, most surgeons feel a postoperative vital capacity of 25% of normal is required in order that the individual does not live a "bed-to-chair" existence. Similarly in the emergency department, patients are generally not felt to be at major risk from an asthma attack until flow rates fall to below about 20% of normal. Individuals with Guillian-Barré syndrome or botulism, in which respiratory muscle weakness can occur, are generally felt to be safe enough to breathe on their own until their ventilation falls below 15 mL/kg (65 mL/kg is normal) *(29)*. Thus, 20–25% of ventilatory function appears adequate to maintain life as well as survive major chest surgery and it therefore follows that if position or weight on the back can cause asphyxiation, the weight applied must be great enough to reduce ventilation below these levels. Furthermore, because it takes several minutes to asphyxiate in the setting of no ventilation, when ventilation is reduced to a lesser extent (between 0 and 25% of normal levels), it will take increasingly longer to asphyxiate.

*THE APPLICATION OF WEIGHT/FORCE*

Currently, there are few data available to rely on concerning the effect of added weight on the back. One study has recently been published that directly addresses the issue of weight on the back and the ventilatory effects of that force. In that study, FVC and $FEV_1$ were compared in the sitting position and in the prone maximal restraint position with 25 pounds and then 50 pounds of weight between the shoulder blades *(30)*. In addition, oxygen saturation and end tidal carbon dioxide ($ETCO_2$) were measured. No significant differences in either $ETCO_2$ or oxygen saturation were noted between either the maximal restraint prone position and sitting, or the maximal restraint prone position with weight on the back (either 25 pounds or 50 pounds). Compared to the maximal restraint prone position, the addition of 25 pounds of weight to the back reduced the FVC by 3% and the addition of 50 pounds of weight further reduced the FVC by another 4%. In a similar fashion, the $FEV_1$ was also reduced. Compared to the maximal restraint prone position, 25 pounds of weight between the shoulder blades reduced the $FEV_1$ by 5% and the addition of 50 pounds reduced the $FEV_1$ by an additional 4%. In *vacuo,* such changes are barely outside the range of normal for these parameters, and therefore they would not be expected to produce any clinically relevant effects.

Studies currently underway in our laboratory would indicate that 225 pounds uniformly distributed over the back only reduces MVV to about 60% of predicted *(31)*. Such relatively small incremental changes with increasing amounts of weight on the back should be expected. Maximal inspiratory pressure is one of the best parameters to measure in order to assess the ability of an individual to move gas (ventilate). The greatest inspiratory pressures are normally generated at lower lung volumes. As an extreme example, the maximal inspiratory pressure an individual can generate at total lung capacity (TLC) is zero and thus as lung volumes are reduced by an external load, it would be expected that the maximal inspiratory pressure that could be generated would increase, tending to preserve spirometric indices as external loads increase.

Furthermore the arguments that weight or force applied to the back limits ventilation to the degree that asphyxiation takes place tend to also rely on the notion that the ventilatory effects of additional body weight are worse in the prone position than in the supine position. Yet our experience in clinical medicine would suggest just the opposite. It is now common practice that when gas exchange is severely impaired because of lung disease, critically ill patients are ventilated in the prone rather than in the supine position *(32–36)*. This evidence from the intensive care unit suggests that the prone position improves gas exchange compared with the supine position. There is now a robust body of clinical research that indicates gas exchange is improved in the prone position and furthermore, it also appears that abdominal distention with upward pressure on the diaphragm improves gas exchange *(37)*. Ward and Macklem have demonstrated that although significant chest wall restriction may impede ventilation, restriction of abdominal motion should not influence ventilatory bellows function because diaphragmatic muscle contraction will occur at a more efficient length in much the same way as higher inspiratory pressures can be generated at low lung volumes *(38)*. Thus, without being able to quantitate the exact effect of weight or force on the back it appears premature to invoke this as a theory to account for these deaths especially in light of the improved gas exchange that appears to occur in this position.

## METABOLIC ACIDOSIS

Still other authors have attempted to invoke "asphyxia" by suggesting that the exertion associated with struggle leads to metabolic acidosis and that restrained individuals are not capable of compensating and normalizing their pH status (by blowing off carbon dioxide) because of the ventilatory impairment occasioned by the restraint position *(39)*. Once again, the data do not support such contentions. Most importantly, even if there were data to support the notion that the hogtie position interfered with ventilation to a degree to cause metabolic acidosis owing to reduced clearance of carbon dioxide in the setting of heavy exercise, the presence of metabolic acidosis does not itself produce asphyxia. As mentioned previously, asphyxia is a process secondary to oxygen deprivation rather than carbon dioxide accumulation or metabolic acidosis. Although it certainly makes individuals uncomfortable, in and of itself the pH generated by even the most intense anaerobic exercise is not dangerous. Perhaps the best example of this in clinical medicine is the physiological effect of a generalized tonic-clonic (grand mal) seizure where significant acidosis can be generated *(40)*.

Moreover, as mentioned earlier, experimental data do not support the contention that the ventilatory response to exercise is in any way blunted by the hogtie position. In a study already cited, individuals were exercised to a mean heart rate of almost 170 beats per minute *(24)*. Following this extremely heavy exercise, they were placed in either a hogtie or sitting position. At the end of 15 minutes in the hogtie position, not only was the $PaO_2$ of individuals in the two groups the same, the $PaCO_2$ was also the same. As $PaCO_2$ is inversely related to alveolar ventilation, the exact same $PaCO_2$ in the two groups indicates that the ventilatory response to exercise in these two groups was exactly the same. Thus, there is no evidence that individuals in the hogtie position ventilate any less than their seated counterparts to any degree. The ventilatory response to the combination of the hogtie position and exercise (and the acidosis associated with exercise) is exactly the same as individuals who exercise and are placed in a seated position.

## OTHER POSITIONS

Despite the overwhelming evidence that the hogtie position is in and of itself not a risk factor for "asphyxia," authors continue to recommend that individuals not be transported in the prone restrained position. Furthermore, they recommend that when an individual requires restraint for transport, he or she should be turned to the side to reduce the risk of "asphyxiation" *(27,39–41)*. Unfortunately, this recommendation is made without regard to the data that do exist. The left and right lateral decubitus position has not been studied recently regarding its effect on ventilation, however, the one study on the subject that does appear in the literature would indicate that vital capacity is affected no more or less in the right or left lateral decubitus position than in the supine position *(42)*. Coupled with the prior work of Vilke, this would indicate that these decubitus positions have basically the same effect on ventilation as does the prone or supine position and that they offer no advantage to these positions *(43)*. In fact, the prone position is to be preferred compared to the supine position for individuals at risk for aspiration. Classically, the supine position is considered the position of greatest risk for an individual whose level of consciousness is depressed and who is at risk of aspiration. Moreover, case reports have documented similar in-custody deaths in individuals who have been placed in the sitting, supine, and lateral restraint positions; thus refuting the supposed greater "safety" from positional or restraint asphyxia in these positions *(39,44)*.

## OTHER FACTORS

Not all authors have accepted the position that restraining an individual in a hogtie or hobble restraint position causes "positional or restraint asphyxia." As noted earlier, Wetli and Fishbain suggested a variety of contributing factors; none of which were asphyxial in nature *(16)*. Laposata stated that the evidence to cite positional asphyxia alone as the cause of death is insufficient and the position "is not itself a position that would be expected to be fatal within minutes" as has been reported in many cases *(45)*. A series of cases from Philadelphia raises the question of whether minor head injury may somehow be related to these deaths, but also points out the well-documented changes in cardiovascular physiology associated with cocaine abuse *(46)*. The authors then go on to state "sudden death during restraint of individuals under the influence of cocaine is most likely the result of these sympathomimetic effects of cocaine." Glatter and Karch applied the "fundamental tenets of basic exercise physiology" to conclude that "the mere act of restraining an agitated individual cannot possibly lead to significant hypoxia (and thus death) unless, of course, there is some preexisting problem with central cardiac output, peripheral oxygen extraction, or oxygen utilization." Using assumptions available in "any basic physiology textbook," they concluded that as "the body has such massive oxygen reserves, and since it has been amply demonstrated that "hog-tying" has only negligible effects on ventilation, we therefore conclude that the diagnosis of "positional asphyxia," by itself, is not a sufficient cause of death, and that other causes for death should be considered" *(47)*.

Recently, a series of sudden deaths in individuals requiring restraint were reported by Stratton *(48)*. This is a retrospective but consecutive study from 1992 to 1998 and represents a series of individuals for whom emergency medical services (EMS) were called and for whom restraint (because of excited delirium) was required. Eighteen deaths occurred in this group and an entrance criterion for the study was that the EMS personnel witnessed the arrest. Factors that were associated with these deaths were then described. As mentioned previously, an entrance criterion for this study was restraint, and therefore, not surprisingly, the authors report that all of the victims were restrained. All were in the prone hobble position, all had a forceful struggle against restraint, and 80% tested positive for stimulants (cocaine, amphetamines, or both). The 18 individuals who died were restrained, with the wrists and ankles bound and attached behind the back. All 196 of the individuals who survived were similarly restrained. Also of note is that for the last 2 years of the study, the position that was recommended for the individuals who were restrained changed. Prior to 1996, patients were restrained in a prone hogtie position. Subsequent to 1996, the less restrictive hobble (also called the total appendage restraint position [TARP]) was used. The death rate while individuals were restrained in the hogtie position was 11%. The death rate remained at 11% after the TARP was adopted.

This is an important study for a variety of reasons. As EMS personnel were on hand and witnessed the arrest, the time between the arrest and the initiation of resuscitative measures must be presumed to be short (although it was not reported). Furthermore, autopsy data concerning the height and heart weight of the individuals were reported for the victims. Analysis of their data reveals that of the 18 individuals, 9 had heart weights that were above 2 standard deviations (SD) from the norm when the height of the individual was used to assess normal heart weight and 2 had heart weights more than 1.5 SD from the norm *(49)*. As only 2.5 % of a normal population will have a heart weight above 2 SD from the norm, the fact that half of this study group was greater than 2 SD, strongly suggests that underlying cardiovascular disease was over-represented in this population. This is not surprising in light of the fact that 45% of this population was reported to have known chronic cocaine use. It is also of note that apparently no cardiac arrests occurred in which there were successful resuscitations. The combination of the presumed short interval between the occurrence of cardiac arrest and resuscitative measures, coupled with the observation that there were no successful resuscitations, strongly suggests that asphyxiation did not play a role in these deaths and that the pathology was predominantly cardiac. This low rate of resuscitation is in keeping with the nationally reported outcomes of cardiac arrests due to heart disease in large cities *(50)*. Finally, the lack of an effect on overall mortality rate by the change in restraint policies in the middle of the study period would also suggest that position had no important effect on the rate of death.

## SUMMARY

Individuals who are out of control and are a risk to either the public or themselves will continue to attract the attention of law enforcement. Because of their behaviors, such individuals are unlikely to readily comply with instructions of either police officers or prehospital personnel. Thus, intervention by the police is almost inevitable. Given the risk of the underlying drugs or exertion that are involved in these situations, it is to be expected that sudden cardiac death may be a consequence of such an interaction. In many respects, such deaths are no more surprising than the death of an individual with occult heart disease shoveling snow after a winter storm. Based on the data that currently exist, the hogtie, maximal restraint position (hobble) or the prone position appear to be no more physiologically disruptive than any other position and insofar as they protect the individual from harming him or herself (e.g., from aspiration) or others, they are, from a medical point of view, perfectly acceptable positions in which to restrain and transport violent and out-of-control individuals. The hypothesis that the maximal restraint position (either hobble or hogtie) in some way places the restrained individual at risk for positional or restraint asphyxiation is not supported by the overwhelming majority of the experimental data that currently exist.

## REFERENCES

1. Reay DT, Eisele JW. Death from law enforcement neck holds. Am J Forensic Med Pathol 1982;3:253–258.
2. Reay DT, Holloway GA Jr. Changes in carotid blood flow produced by neck compression. Am J Forensic Med Pathol 1982;3:199–202.
3. Burgreen B, Krosch C, Binkerd V, Blackbourne B. Final report of the custody death task force. San Diego Police Department, San Diego, CA, 1992.
4. O'Halloran RL, Lewman LV. Restraint asphyxiation in excited delirium. Am J Forensic Med Pathol 1993;14(4):289–295.
5. Stratton SJ, Rogers C, Green K. Sudden death in individuals in hobble restraints during paramedic transport. Ann Emerg Med 1995;25(5):710–712.
6. Reay DT, Fligner CL, Stilwell AD, Arnold J. Positional asphyxia during law enforcement transport. Am J Forensic Med Pathol 1992;13(2):90–97.
7. Bates DV, Macklem PT, Christie RV. Respiratory Function in Disease. WB Saunders, New York, NY, 1971.

8. Astrand PO, Rodahl K. Textbook of Work Physiology McGraw-Hill, New York, NY, 1977, pp. 207-266
9. Bell MD, Rao VJ, Wetli CV, Rodriguez RN. Positional asphyxiation in adults: a series of 30 cases from the Dade and Broward county Florida medical examiner offices from 1982–1990. Am J Forensic Med Path 1992;13(2):101–107.
10. Dube AH, Mitchell EK. Accidental strangulation from vest restraints. JAMA 1986;256(19):2725–2726.
11. Katz L. Accidental strangulation from vest restrants. JAMA 1987;257(15): 2032–2033.
12. Di Maio VJM, Dana SE, Bux RC. Deaths caused by restraint vests. JAMA 1986;256(7):905.
13. Miles S. A case of death by physical restraint: new lessons from a photograph. J Am Geriatrics Soc 1996;44:291–292.
14. Miles HS, Irvine P. Deaths caused by physical restraints. Gerontologist 1992;32:762–726.
15. Emson HE. Death in a restraint jacket from mechanical asphyxia. Can Med Assoc J 1994;151(7):985–987.
16. Wetli CV, Fishbain DA. Cocaine-induced psychosis and sudden death in recreational cocaine users. J Forensic Sci 1985;30(3):873–880.
17. Ross DL. An analysis of in-custody deaths and positional asphyxiation. The Police Marksman 1996;March/April:16–18.
18. Reay DT, Howard JD, Fligner CL, Ward RJ. Effects of positional restraint on oxygen saturation and heart rate following exercise. Am J Forensic Med Pathol 1988;9(1):16–18.
19. Levitzky MG. Pulmonary Physiology, 4th ed. McGraw-Hill, New York, NY, 1995.
20. Wasserman K, Hansen JE, Sue DY, Whipp BJ, Casburi R. Normal values. In: Wasserman K, Hansen JE, Sue DY, Whipp BJ, Casaburi R, eds. Principles of Exercise Testing and Interpretation, 2nd ed. Lea & Febiger, Philadelphia, PA,1994, pp. 127–128.
21. Biebuyck JF. Pulse oximetry. Anesthesiology 1989;70:98–108.
22. Norton LH, Squires B, Craig NP, et al. Accuracy of pulse oximetry during exercise stress testing. Int J Sports Med 1992;13:523–527.
23. Hansen JE, Casaburi R. Validity of ear oximetry in clinical exercise testing. Chest 1987;91(3):333.
24. Chan TC, Vilke GM, Neuman T, Clausen JL. Restraint position and positional asphyxia. Ann Emerg Med Ann Emerg Med 1997;30(5):578–586.
25. Schmidt MA, Snowden T, Clin J. The effects of positional restraint on oxygen saturation and heart rate. J Emerg Med 1999;17(5):777–782.
26. Chan TC, Vilke GM, Clausen J, Clark RF, Schmidt P, Snowden T, Neuman T. The effect of oleoresin capsicum "pepper" spray inhalation on respiratory function. J Forensic Sci 2002;47(2):28–33.
27. Parkes J. Sudden death during restraint. A study to measure restraint positions on the rate of recovery from exercise. Med Sci Law 2000;40(1):39–44.

28. Reay DT. Death in custody. Clinics in Lab Med 1998;18(1):1–22.
29. Rochester DF, Esau SA. The respiratory muscles. In: Baum GL, Wolinsky E. eds. A Textbook of Pulmonary Diseases. Little Brown, Boston, MA, 1994.
30. Chan TC, Neuman T, Clausen J, Eisele J, Vilke GM. Weight force during prone restraint and respiratory function. Am J Forensic Med Pathol 2004;25:185–189.
31. Vilke GM, Michalewicz B, Kohlkorst F, Neuman T, Chan TC. Does weight force during physical restraint cause respiratory compromise? Acad Emerg Med 2005;12(5):16.
32. Mure M, Martling CR, Lindahl SGE. Dramatic effect on oxygenation in patients with severe acute lung insufficiency treated in the prone position Crit Care Med 1997;25(9):1539–1544.
33. Douglas WW, Rehder K, Beynen FM, Sessler AD, Marsh HM. Improved oxygenation in patients with acute respiratory failure: the prone position. ARRD 1977;115:559–566.
34. Albert RK. The prone position in acute respiratory distress syndrome: where we are, and where do we go from here. Crit Care Med 1997;25(9):1453–1454.
35. Langer M, Mascheroni D, Marcolin R, Gattinoni L. The prone position in ARDS. Patients Chest 1988;94(1):103–107.
36. Piehl MA, Brown RS. Use of extreme position changes in acute respiratory failure. Crit. Care Med 1976; 4(1):13–14.
37. Mure M, Glenny RW, Domino KB, Hlastala MP. Pulmonary gas exchange improves in the prone position with abdominal distention. Am J Resp Crit Care Med 1998;157:1785–1790.
38. Ward M, Macklem PT. The act of breathing and how it fails. Chest 1990;97(3):36S–39S.
39. Hick JL, Smith SW, Lynch MT. Metabolic acidosis in restraint associated cardiac arrest: a case series. Acad. Emerg. Med 1999;6(3):239–243.
40. Stratton SJ, Rogers C, Green K. Sudden death in individuals in hobble restraints during paramedic transport. Ann Emerg Med 1995;25:710–712.
41. Reay DT. Suspect restraint and sudden death. FBI Law Enforcement Bulletin May 22-25, 1996.
42. Kaneko K, Milic-Emili J, Dolovich MB, Dawson A, Bates DV. Regional distribution of ventilation and perfusion as a function of body position. J Appl Physiol 1966;21(3):767–777.
43. Vilke GM, Chan TC, Neuman T, Clausen JL. Spirometry in normal subjects in sitting, prone, and supine positions. Respir Care 2000;45(4):407–410.
44. Kupas DF, Wydro GC. Patient restraint in emergency medical services systems. Prehosp Emerg Care 2002;6:340–345.
45. Laposata EA. Positional asphyxia during law enforcement transport (Letter). Am J Forensic Med Pathol 1993;14:86.
46. Mirchandani HG, Rorke LB, Sekula-Perlman A, Hood IC. Cocaine-induced agitated delirium, forceful struggle, and minor head injury. Am J Forensic Med Pathol 1994;15(2):95–99.

47. Glatter K, Karch SB. Positional asphyxia: inadequate oxygen, or inadequate theory? Forensic Sci Intern 2004;141:201–202.
48. Stratton SJ, Rogers C, Brickett K, Gruzinski G. Factors associated with sudden death of individuals requiring restraint for excited delerium. Amer J Emerg Med 2001;19:187–191.
49. Zeck PM. The weight of the normal heart. Arch Pathol 1942;34:820–832.
50. Becker LB, Ostrander MP, Barrett J, Kondos GT. Outcome of CPR in a large metropolitan area-Where are the survivors? Ann Emerg Med 1991;20:355–361.

# Chapter 5

# Restraint Stress

## Elizabeth A. Laposata

### INTRODUCTION

How can death during police restraint be explained when the pathologist finds no structural or anatomic lesions to explain death? This is not an easy question to answer. When an in-custody restraint death occurs, there is a close physical and temporal association between the restraint process and the death that follows. Because of this, it is tempting to attribute the cause of death to the restraint procedure itself. However, this is an error of logic: the fallacy of *post hoc ergo propter hoc*, which is Latin for "after this therefore because of this." This error in logic may mislead death investigators into building a case centered on the deadly effects of police restraint procedures and prevent consideration of other mechanisms and causes of death that occur contemporaneous with restraint. One such cause is cardiorespiratory arrest caused by the acute stress response occurring during police restraint. This cause of sudden death is unpredictable and rare, and results from a combination of individual perception of the threat posed by the restraint events and maladaptive pathophysiology of the acute stress response. This chapter examines the mechanisms, physiology, and medical issues associated with the acute stress response.

### HISTORY

Historically, the modern medical concept of stress evolved from observations of fear linked to unexplained death. In 1897, Walter Bradford Cannon, one of America's leading physiologists, noticed that when his experimental animals

From: *Forensic Science and Medicine: Sudden Deaths in Custody*
Edited by: D. L. Ross and T. C. Chan © Humana Press Inc., Totowa, NJ

were frightened or in some other way disturbed, peristaltic waves in the stomach sometimes ceased abruptly *(1)*. This finding led him to investigate the effects of emotions on physiological processes. Cannon showed that strong arousal in an animal caused stimulation of the sympathetic division of the autonomic nervous system to combine with release of large amounts of the hormone adrenaline, which he called "sympathin" (later identified as a mixture of epinephrine and norepinephrine), which mobilizes the animal for an emergency response of "fight or flight" *(2)*. Cannon documented that this response caused physiological changes, such as increases in blood sugar level, pulse rate, and blood pressure, and diversion of blood flow to the skeletal muscles. He concluded that these physiological responses, the so-called "sympathico-adrenal system," were responsible for marshaling resources to respond to a threat with a "violent display of energy" *(1)*.

Case studies illustrating Cannon's hypothesis were first published in his classic reference *Voodoo Death*, which appeared in the *American Anthropologist* in 1942 *(3)*. A voodoo death, as defined by Cannon, is the sudden, medically unexplained death resulting from a voodoo curse. Studying the records of anthropologists and missionaries who lived among natives of South America, Africa, Haiti, Australia, New Zealand, and the Islands of the Pacific, Cannon found accounts of death induced by fright after men were condemned by their medicine man or chief. Paulino Soares de Sousa (1807–1866) was the first to report that in Brazil the medicine man of the Tupinambas Indians could cause death induced by fright by condemning a member of the community. The book, *New Zealand and Its Aborigines,* published in 1845 contains an account of a woman who ate some fruit taken from a tabooed place. When she was told, she lamented and was convinced that the spirit of the place would kill her. Within 24 hours, she was dead *(4)*. Cannon hypothesized from this and other case reports that a persistent state of fear can cause death. He tied his knowledge of physiology to these reports of voodoo death and concluded that intense action of the sympathico-adrenal system could have lethal results, especially if the organism was denied the ability to act and resolve the situation. However, he never applied the term "stress" to these events.

In the 1950s, Hans Selye introduced the concept of the stress syndrome as a medical entity in his book, *The Physiology and Pathology of Exposure to Stress (5)*. He documented enlargement of the adrenal cortex, gastrointestinal ulceration, and thymicolymphatic involution in experimental animals exposed to a wide variety of harmful physical stimuli *(6)*. Selye's concept of a stress syndrome included the secretion of hormones from the adrenal cortex in response to environmental events.

Selye also introduced the term *general adaptation syndrome*, which divided the nonspecific response of the body to any demand placed on it into three phases. Phase 1 was an alarm reaction where the body's resources were mobilized; phase 2 was resistance, where the body tried to cope with the stressor; and, finally, phase 3 was exhaustion, where physiological reserves were depleted *(7)*. During these phases, Selye hypothesized that the intensity of the response might vary but it would always involve the same neurological and endocrine patterns.

In the late 1960s, Holmes and Rahe introduced the social re-adjustment scale, which documented that these physiological responses can occur in the modern everyday world *(8)*. This scale is a list of life events that are associated with varying degrees of stress-response physiology in the individual going through the specific experience. Holmes and Rahe found the most stressful life experience to be death of a spouse, followed by divorce or separation, and, interestingly enough, then detention in jail. Thus, being in jail or the perception of going to jail, may precipitate the onset of stress physiology in some individuals.

What then accounts for different individual responses to the same stressful life event? In 1984, Lazarus introduced the term *stress appraisal*. According to Lazarus, what matters is not the actual event, but how the individual perceives and interprets the event *(9)*. This process of perceiving and interpreting the event is called appraisal. Thus, stress is a very personal physiological response, depending not so much on the event itself, but on how the individual perceives and interprets the event. Two people exposed to the same exact events may perceive and interpret them differently, and, therefore, each may have a different physiological response.

In the mid-1990s, Blascovich and Tomaka developed the biopsychosocial model of stress *(10)*. This model brought together the stress physiology and biology defined by Cannon and Selye with the psychosocial stressors as defined by Holmes and Lazarus. Blascovich and Tomaka proposed that three items determined the magnitude of stress: the individual's internal environment or physiology, the external environment, and the dynamics of the interaction between the two. As stress increased from what they termed a "challenge" to a "threat," the sympathetic–adrenal–medulla (SAM) axis would be activated first, followed by the hypothalamic–pituitary–adrenal (HPA) axis. Thus, the perception of an increasingly severe stressful situation would serve to recruit additional neuroendocrine responses, possibly to the detriment of the individual mounting that response.

Stress can be understood as a negative emotional experience accompanied by predictable biochemical, psychological, cognitive, and behavioral changes

**Table 1**
**Physiological Results of the Acute Stress Response**

- Increased arterial blood pressure
- Increased blood flow to active skeletal muscles
- Increased muscle strength
- Increased cellular metabolic rate
- Increased blood glucose
- Increased glycolysis in liver and muscles
- Increased tolerance to pain

that are directed at preparing the individual to either alter the stressful event (i.e., fight) or accommodate to it (i.e., flight). A similar environmental stimulus may cause a full cascade of neuroendocrine biochemical events in one person and not in another because of the individual's perception of the situation. As first reported in voodoo deaths, physiological responses produced by the individual's perception of his or her environment can cause death without the presence of any physical injury.

## PHYSIOLOGICAL CHANGES ASSOCIATED WITH THE ACUTE STRESS RESPONSE

A cascade of neuroendocrine events produces the physiological changes of the acute stress response. The neuroendocrine response to stress is a biological reaction triggered by sudden changes in the social or physical environment in order to give the individual the greatest chances for survival (Table 1). Once the individual recognizes stress, hormones from the pituitary and adrenal glands enter the blood, initiating a complex cascade of physiological responses and regulation feedback loops. From the pituitary, these include adrenocorticotropic hormone (ACTH), β-endorphin, prolactin, growth hormone, and vasopressin. The adrenal contributions are cortisol, epinephrine, and norepinephrine. Both psychological and physical stresses cause the same neuroendocrine responses *(11,12)*.

The most proximal element in the neuroendocrine response cascade is the hypothalamus. The hypothalamus activates two cascades: the adrenal medulla (SAM axis) via the brainstem, spinal cord, and splanchnic nerves and the pituitary gland (HPA axis) via the hypothalamohypophysial portal circulation (Fig. 1).

### Sympathetic–Adrenal–Medulla Axis

Neurons in the hypothalamus traverse one relay station in the brainstem, then these preganglionic sympathetic nerve fibers pass without synapsing via

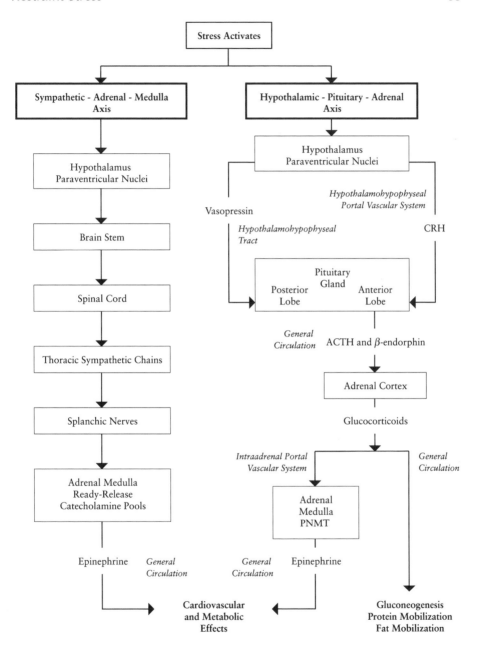

**Fig. 1.** The neuroendocrine cascade of the acute stress response.

the interomediolateral horn of the spinal cord through the sympathetic chains, through the splanchnic nerves (T7–T11), to the adrenal medulla. Once in the adrenal medulla, this innervation stimulates synthesis and release of catecholamines from the adrenal medulla chromaffin cells. The chromaffin adrenal medullary cells contain a "ready release pool" of catecholamines (80% epinephrine and 20% norepinephrine), which is discharged upon stimulation, followed by discharge of a so-called slow-release pool *(13)*. The timing for release of both of these pools, however, is on the order of microseconds. The circulating epinephrine and norepinephrine have almost the same effects on their target organs as direct sympathetic stimulation except that their effects last 5 to 10 times longer because these hormones are removed slowly from the blood. Norepinephrine is also released into the systemic circulation from spillover from sympathetic nerve stimulation *(14)*.

The physiological activation of the "fight-or-flight response can be preceded by a so-called mental anticipatory phase *(15)*. The significance of this anticipatory phase is that it activates the adrenal medulla by translocating the reserve pool of catecholamine granules into the rapidly releasable pool. Hence, stimulation of the SAM axis following anticipation results in secretion of a larger number of granules and, potentially, extraordinarily high plasma catecholamine concentrations. High catecholamine levels may explain the phenomena of stress-induced analgesia, where the perception of pain is blunted, and of markedly increased muscle strength sometimes noted as part of the acute stress response *(16)*.

Epinephrine, acting through $\alpha$- and $\beta$-receptors, has cardiovascular and metabolic actions *(17,18)*. Cardiovascular effects activated by $\alpha$-1 and $\alpha$-2 adrenergic receptors increase systemic vascular resistance and arterial pressure. $\beta$-Receptors have positive chronotropic and inotrophic effects, increasing heart rate and myocardial contractility. Thus, myocardial oxygen consumption and energy demands are also increased. Epinephrine has many metabolic actions including increasing blood glycerol, free fatty acids, glucose, lactate, and $\beta$-hydroxybutyrate. Epinephrine secreted by the adrenal medulla can increase the metabolic rate of the body as much as 100% above normal.

Occasionally, the effects of epinephrine on heart rate, metabolic rate, blood lactate, and blood glucose have been noted to persist long after the threat stimulus has been removed *(19)*. Persistent cellular effects of epinephrine in tissue after blood levels have returned to normal or the unexpected persistence of high blood levels of epinephrine may explain this effect. For example, after cessation of strenuous exercise, epinephrine levels may still be elevated 2 hours later in some individuals *(20)*. Thus, the "depo-effect" may explain the delayed appearance or unexpected persistence of epinephrine toxic actions.

## Hypothalamic–Pituitary–Adrenocortical Axis

The HPA axis meets the demands of stress primarily through the synthesis and release of three key hormones: corticotropin-releasing hormone (CRH), ACTH, and cortisol *(21)*. Neurons of the paraventricular nucleus of the hypothalamus synthesize CRH in response to stress stimuli. CRH then travels down the axons of these neurons to the external layer of the median eminence where it is released into the portal circulation to reach the anterior pituitary. The anterior pituitary cells (pituitary corticotrophs) then release ACTH. Many of the CRH-containing neurons of the paraventricular nucleus of the hypothalamus also release vasopressin. Vasopressin secreted by the hypothalamus potentates the ability of CRH to promote ACTH release from the pituitary upon exposure to stress *(22)*. In addition to releasing ACTH upon CRH stimulation, the pituitary gland releases β-endorphins. This may explain the finding that CRH administration in humans has been shown to alter attention, mood, and to decrease pain perception *(23)*.

ACTH released into the general circulations acts on the adrenal cortex stimulating it to produce glucocorticoids, mineralocorticoids, and adrenal androgens. The glucocorticoids are synthesized from precursor cholesterol in the zona fasciculata/reticularis of the adrenal cortex. They enter the medullary area of the adrenal gland via sinusoidal blood. The cortisol from the adrenal cortex induces phenylethanolamine-$N$-methyl transferase (PNMT) in the medulla, the rate-limiting enzyme responsible for the conversion of norepinephrine to epinephrine. The glucocorticoids then enter the general circulation via the medullary veins of the adrenal glands. An important consequence of the release of glucocorticoids into the blood is the elevation of blood glucose to provide fuel for the increased metabolic demands of the stress response *(24)*.

Thus, the acute stress response is a complex cascade of interactions between the central and autonomic nervous system, endocrine hormone secretion, and end-organ responses to enable an individual to survive (i.e., to fight or flee). Because of the complexity of these stress cascades and depending on the individual's threat appraisal, it is not surprising that stress responses of an organism are neither identical, predictable, nor consistently reproducible.

## RESTRAINT AND THE ACUTE STRESS RESPONSE

In 1936, Selye was the first researcher to use immobilization as a model for the stress response *(25)*. Selye's original restraint procedure involved tying a rat's legs together, then wrapping the rat in a towel. When repeatedly applied, this restraint in rats led to manifestations of what Selye termed the general adaptation response to stress consisting of adrenal hypertrophy, gastric ulceration, and thymicolymphatic involution.

Furthermore, neuroanatomical and neurophysiological laboratory studies indicate that different types of stressors have different neuronal circuits that comprise their own unique, so-called "signatures" *(7)*. Techniques for studying the stress response and elucidating the particular pathways include intracerebral microdialysis, immunohistochemistry, track-tracing techniques, and *in situ* hybridization for neurotransmitters, neuropeptides, and proto-oncogenes. By studying *c-Fos* immunoreactivity, paraventricular nuclear extracellular norepinephrine levels, amygdala norepinephrine levels, and plasma levels of various hormones, five models of central neuroendocrine stress-related "signatures" have been characterized: pain, hemorrhage, hypoglycemia, cold, and immobilization *(7)*.

Using immobilization, Kubo et al. studied the central mechanisms controlling stress-induced increased blood pressure *(26)*. Their model produced stress by putting a rat in a small cylindrical devise (6.5 cm × 15 cm) that held each rat at a normal standing position. Because stimulation of the amygdala was known to increase blood pressure, they examined the activity of neurons in the amygdala by studying the expression of *c-Fos*. *C-Fos* is a gene that produces a protein (called c-Fos) that activates DNA transcription and causes cell activation. Therefore, the amount of c-Fos protein detected immunohistochemically is a reflection of general cell activation. They found that in rats that had been restrained, the number of neurons in the medial amygdaloid nucleus that showed c-Fos immunoreactivity increased compared with nonrestrained rats. This increase in neuronal activity correlated with increased blood pressure *(26)*.

In other studies, acute stress response to restraint was induced by taping each limb of a rat to a metal frame and keeping the rat in the prone position. Strong *c-Fos* activation was observed in several regions in the brain after this immobilization stress, indicating that numerous neuronal circuits were activated. These included brainstem catecholaminergic nuclei involved in cardiorespiratory control, noncatecholaminergic nuclei involved in temperature regulation, midline thalamic nuclei, hypothalamus, amygdala, and neurons in the parietal somatosensory cerebral cortex *(27,28)*. Acute immobilization stress also increased levels of CRH mRNA, and vasopressin mRNA in the paraventricular nucleus of the thalamus *(29,30)*.

In reviewing some 500 neurophysiological studies of stress, Pacak et al. proposed that specific neuronal circuits and pathways were activated by immobilization stress *(7,17)*. Ascending pathways to the hypothalamic paraventricular nucleus started with somatosensory neurons from the periphery ascending the spinoreticular tracts to the brainstem. In the brainstem, ventral noradrenergic and noncatecholaminergic pathways then connected to the hypothalamus. The descending limb of the stress pathway arose from cortical, limbic, hypothalamic, and some brainstem nuclei and then connected to motor and autonomic, central, and peripheral neurons.

In addition to neural pathways, the effect of stress on biochemistry in the adrenal gland has also been studied using the restraint model of acute stress *(31)*. The acute stress response in immobilized rats caused glucocorticoids produced in the adrenal cortex to enter the intra-adrenal portal vascular system and deliver a high concentration of glucocorticoids to the adrenal medulla. These high concentrations induced PNMT mRNA synthesis and subsequent synthesis of the enzyme responsible for the conversion of norepinephrine to epinephrine *(32)*.

In addition to producing a laboratory model to study the stress physiology, restraint without physical injury has been reported to cause death in animals from so-called fear paralysis. The fear paralysis reflex in animals is characterized by immediate, profound bradycardia that proceeds to asystole. Death has been observed to occur in wild rats simply being held tightly. The reflex bradycardia may be the consequence of carotid body stimulation by stress-induced increases in arterial pressure. Restraint of movement is one of the most powerful stimuli to induce this fear paralysis and death in animals *(16,33)*.

Thus, restraint is a laboratory model of the acute stress response and has been used to study the neuroendocrine and physiological effects of stress. Because laboratory studies document that the acute stress response occurs in animals during restraint procedures, by extension, it is likely that the acute stress response can occur in individuals who are restrained by police.

## INDIVIDUAL PERCEPTION AND THE ACUTE STRESS RESPONSE

Individual perception is a key factor in producing the acute stress response to restraint. The acute stress response to restraint is specifically programmed into the hardware of living organisms. However, individual perception can determine whether an event, such as restraint, produces the acute stress response. Whether one perceives a situation as a threat, either psychological or physical, is crucial in determining whether the fight-or-flight physiological response will occur. Factors involved in setting the threshold for stress recognition have not been precisely defined and vary from individual to individual.

In the 1960s, Lazarus conducted pioneering studies that defined the importance of the thought process in appraisal of events in producing the negative emotions associated with the stress response *(10)*. He measured the physiological stress responses in individuals who viewed a threatening film depicting woodshop-related accidents. One group received instruction about viewing the upcoming film so group members would understand what was going to take place (i.e., intellectualization). The other group had no such instruction. Physiological indicators of the acute stress reaction during the film, such as increased heart rate and electrodermal skin conductance, were lower for the group that had more control over its situation by having intellectual information about what they were going to see. Thus, he showed that how an individual thinks about and evaluates a noxious stimulus determines the nature of the emotional and physiological responses that follow.

Athletic competition is another example where one can see the role that perception plays in determining physiological stress responses. More pronounced endocrine changes have been reported in track and field athletes after an international race compared with a national race of identical duration and intensity of muscular work. This is owing to the difference in psychological stress of the events, even though the physical stress is the same *(34)*.

The individual perception also influences being able to shut off the response when the threat has passed. For example, most people initially react to the challenge of public speaking by activation of the HPA axis, causing increased heart rate, blood pressure, and cortisol levels. After repeated public speaking, however, most people become habituated, no longer perceiving the event as stressful, and their cortisol secretion no longer increases with the challenge. However, approximately 10% of those subjects studied continue to perceive public speaking as stressful, and their cortisol levels increased each time they spoke in public. The innate factors that account for these differences are unknown *(35)*.

The relationship between the perception of an event as stressful and sudden cardiac death is clearly recognized in the cardiology literature. Acute mental stress has been shown to lead to acute sinus tachycardia, hypertension, and a high degree of cardiac electrical instability *(36)*. In patients with acute coronary syndromes, Reich et al. noted that anger was a trigger for up to 15% of life-threatening dysrhythmias *(37)*. Varieur and Mittlemen "attribute the lethal effects of anger in some circumstances to its activation of high-gain central-neural circuitry in the sympathetic nervous system leading to myocardial electrical instability," that is, the acute stress response *(36)*.

It is difficult to assess the impact of an external event on an individual. Theoretically, one can predict what the consequences of an event are likely to

### Table 2
### Effects of Epinephrine

| Adaptive | | Maladaptive |
|---|---|---|
| **Cardiovascular** | | |
| • Increased chronotropic and inotropic effects | • β-receptors | • dysrhythmias and myocardial ischemia |
| • Increased systemic vascular resistance | • α-1 & α-2 receptors | • reflex bradycardia and pulmonary edema |
| • Increased arterial pressure | | |
| **Metabolic** | | |
| • Increased glucose availability especially in liver and skeletal muscles | • Activates cellular phosphorylase | • Lactic acidosis |
| • Chemical thermogenesis | • Increases rate of cellular metabolism | • Hyperthermia |

be in a large number of individuals, but we remain unsure about how to predict the effects on any one individual in particular. Because the same environmental events produce different responses in different individuals and, indeed different responses at different times in the same individual, the distinguishing feature of stress becomes the behavioral response rather than the situation in which it occurs *(38)*. Furthermore, anticipation of the event, so-called anticipatory stress, can start the preparation for secretion of mediators like CRH, cortisol, and epinephrine prior to the actual stressful event taking place *(15,35)*. Thus, predicting who will perceive a restraint procedure in a way that triggers the acute stress response with the risk for sudden unexpected death is not clear.

## FACTORS IN SUDDEN DEATH DURING THE ACUTE STRESS RESPONSE

### Role of Epinephrine

Epinephrine is a key effector of physiological changes caused by the neuroendocrine stress cascade. However, in addition to its positive adaptive effects, epinephrine can produce fatal cardiac, pulmonary, and metabolic side effects (Table 2). Epinephrine can induce fatal cardiac dysrhythmias that are unpredictable in their occurrence *(39,40)*. In addition to the acute stress response, epinephrine levels are also increased by exercise and hypoxia *(20,41)*. Thus, the combination of struggle (i.e., exercise and increased oxygen demands), and the acute stress response that occur during police restraint procedures can increase epinephrine levels even higher and potentially enhance its toxic effects. Epinephrine-induced increases in arterial blood pressure can also trigger baroreceptors located in the carotid body that relay impulses to the medullary vagal center. Increased vagal tone causes bradycardia that may progress to asystole. In addition to the lethal dysrhythmias, high levels of epinephrine may produce pulmonary edema and impair oxygenation. Experimentally, epinephrine administration is used to produce a reproducible model of pulmonary edema *(42)*.

Epinephrine can also cause life-threatening metabolic lactic acidosis because of the elevation of lactic acid as a byproduct of anaerobic glycolysis following epinephrine-induced increases in oxidative metabolism. Lactic acidosis has been reported in patients who received epinephrine as a vasopressor agent after coronary artery bypass graft surgery *(43)*. In addition, lactic acidosis developed when an intravenous drug user inadvertently injected 20 mg of epinephrine intravenously *(44)*. Importantly, lactic acidosis has been reported in cases of sudden death occurring during police restraint *(45,46)*. Thus, some restraint-associated cardiac arrests may be explained by these metabolic side effects of epinephrine.

Although epinephrine is usually cleared quickly after release with a half-life of 1 to 2 minutes, the removal of the stimulus does not always result in the rapid return of plasma levels of epinephrine to baseline concentrations. This phenomenon as described on p. 64 is known as the "depo-effect" *(19)*. Continued epinephrine-induced changes in heart rate and basal metabolic rate may explain sudden death after restraint procedures are accomplished and the detainee appears calm.

Thus, the physiological consequences of the actions of epinephrine may cause sudden unexpected death during the acute stress response to restraint. These are functional effects that do not cause anatomic or structural changes in the body. The result may be the so-called autopsy-negative death or a death without anatomic findings sufficient to explain death.

## *Role of Drug-Induced or Psychiatric Manic States*

Psychotic states, either naturally occurring psychiatric disease or drug-induced psychosis, can increase the risk of sudden death during the acute stress response during restraint. Use of cocaine can cause a manic state, agitated delirium, that shares some of the same physiological mechanisms as those produced by the fight-or-flight acute stress response (*see* Chapters 6 and 7). Sudden death in these cocaine users can occur unpredictably, either with or without police restraint *(47–49)*.

Agitation caused by manic and/or paranoid psychiatric illness is also a risk for sudden death during restraint owing to recruitment of the same neuroendocrine cascades as the acute stress response *(50,51)*. Because individual perception of a situation is the trigger for the HPA and SAM cascades, an individual with a mental state altered by disease or drugs may perceive a threat in what is, in reality, a situation that is not life-threatening. This misperception of reality could be strengthened by police intervention while trying to take an individual into custody, thus reinforcing the apparent reality of a paranoid or psychotic state.

## Role of Heart Disease

Cardiovascular diseases can decrease the threshold for an adverse outcome to the acute stress response. Patients with minimal atherosclerotic coronary artery disease can develop angina and electrocardiographic (ECG) manifestations of ischemia when undergoing psychological stress or when given epinephrine *(40)*. Increases in cortisol and catecholamines increase coronary artery tone and decrease the blood flow reduction already produced by fixed minimal stenosis *(40,52)*. Thus, at postmortem examination, the minimal atherosclerotic coronary artery stenosis may cause myocardial ischemia and dysrhythmias during the acute stress response, especially when combined with the increased myocardial energy demands of physical exertion.

Individuals with hypertension may have a potentially increased risk of death during the stress response. Experimental studies in animals have shown that spontaneously hypertensive rats and mice are more reactive to stress than their normotensive counterparts *(53)*. Furthermore, immobilization leads to greater changes in heart rate, blood pressure, and body temperature in the hypertensive rodents than in the normotensive ones.

Patients with prolonged corrected QT intervals on ECG are at risk for sudden death during stressful events. Adrenergic stimulation of cardiac electric activity is thought to be critical for triggering potentially malignant dysrhythmias, such as ventricular tachycardia, ventricular fibrillation, and torsades de pointes, which can lead to sudden death *(54)*. Prolonged QT syndromes can be either congenital or acquired. There are two forms of the hereditary syndrome: the Jervell Lange-Nielson syndrome and the Romano Ward syndrome. The prolonged QT is associated with deafness in the Jervell Lange-Nielsen syndrome; in the Romano Ward syndrome hearing is normal. Observations of what is now considered the Jervell Lange-Nielsen syndrome date back to a case report in 1856 that describes a deaf child who experienced sudden cardiac death while being admonished at school. Two of her siblings had also died suddenly after episodes of fright *(55)*.

A prolonged QT interval can be acquired by the administration of certain drugs or by the presence of disease. Drugs that may prolong the QT interval include antipsychotics, tricyclic antidepressants, some antibiotics and antifungals, calcium channel blockers, and antiretroviral agents *(56,57)*. Factors not related to drugs that may prolong the QT interval include electrolyte disturbances, such as low potassium and magnesium, heart failure, and myocardial ischemia. Although the absolute risk of development of prolonged QT and life-threatening dysrhythmias is probably extremely low when a single QT-prolonging drug or condition is present, the risk, however, may be more significant when several factors are combined.

## Role of Personal History

The interpretation of what is or is not a threat to an individual is based in part on prior experiences, developmental history, and genetic predisposition. In animal models, the vulnerability of many systems of the body to stress is influenced by experiences early in life. In rats, unpredictable prenatal stress caused increased reactivity of the HPA axis and sympathetic nervous system. These effects lasted throughout the animal's life span. Conversely, routine gentle handling of postnatal rats counteracted the effects of prenatal stress and resulted in reduced reactivity of the HPA axis and sympathetic nervous system *(58)*. These types of studies suggest that in humans, prenatal adverse conditions and early life events, such as parental behavior, may exert long-lasting influences on the neuroendocrine stress response. Once the reactivity of the hypothalamic–pituitary axis and adrenocortical systems is established by deleterious events early in life, the subsequent functioning of these cascades in adult life may be maladaptive.

A few animal studies have investigated the genomic contribution to the stress response using genetic analysis (quantitative trait locus analysis) *(59)*. Using changes in body temperature as a marker of stress during immobilization, two trait loci were found in the rat model. This suggests the possibility of genetic determinates of reactivity to stress. Furthermore, in humans, genetic polymorphisms have been found that influence β-adrenergic stimulation and could determine the vascular response to stress *(60)*. The understanding of genomic pathways leading to pathological levels of stress response may someday have the potential for identifying individuals with pathological susceptibility to stress.

## Role of Chronic Stress and Conditioning

The overlay of an acute stress reaction on chronic stress changes the magnitude of the acute stress response *(21)*. Chronic stress induces sustained CRH release from the paraventricular nuclei of the hypothalamus. On this baseline, any response to an acute stress episode is enhanced. Pituitary vasopressin receptors increase in chronic stress. Vasopressin may become a regulator along with CRH to mediate the hyper-responsiveness of the hypothalamic–pituitary axis in chronic stress. Thus, the level of chronic stress that an individual is under may affect the level of physiological response to an acute stressor.

There are other modifiers of response to acute stress such as age, race, diet, and physical conditioning. Johansson and Ake studied cardiovascular reactivity to adrenergic agonists in response to mental stress and exercise *(61)*. Younger subjects were more sensitive to the adrenergic agonists resulting in higher heart rates than middle-aged subjects. This suggests that the older subjects may have decreased β-adrenergic responsiveness. The dietary intake of sodium has also been studied for its effect on cardiovascular response to psychological stressors. Heart rate and blood pressure responses to mental stress testing were compared before and after 14 days of high dietary sodium intake. The increased dietary sodium intake increased the blood pressure responses during mental stress in individuals with a family history of hypertension but not in those without *(24)*. Thus, increased dietary intake of sodium may increase peripheral vascular resistance to psychological stressors in certain individuals. In the model of the spontaneously hypertensive rat, responses to environmental stressors were accentuated after a high-sodium diet compared to hypertensive rats without a high-sodium diet. Surprisingly, physical conditioning had little effect on the neuroendocrine response to stressors *(62)*.

## ACUTE STRESS RESPONSE AND SUDDEN DEATH DURING RESTRAINT

Unexpected sudden death during restraint procedures may be the result of the acute stress response and not because of any damaging physical effects of the restraint procedures themselves. This concept is consistent with what is known about the risk for death intrinsic to the neuroendocrine acute stress response that can be triggered by being restrained. Sudden death from the acute stress response during restraint can occur unpredictably and, indeed, rarely considering how often restraint procedures are used with no ill effects. To prepare the animal for fight or escape, the neuroendocrine cascades allow for complex types of responses in many different organs. Modifiers that are unique to the individual can further alter these responses. In addition, in humans, the acute stress response may be triggered by psychological factors based on the individual's perception of the events.

Death during the acute stress response induced by restraint procedures has also been reported in settings other than police settings. These deaths, however, generally do not receive the intense media attention and public scrutiny that accompany deaths in police custody.

Case reports in the geriatric medical literature link death of elderly during restraint procedures to the significant psychological stress of forced immobilization leading to the acute stress response, ventricular dysrhythmias, and sudden death *(63,64)*. In psychiatric settings, patients suffering from excited delirium or other manic psychosis while being restrained in medically supervised and prescribed ways may still suffer sudden unexpected cardiorespiratory arrests *(50,51)*.

A survey of the literature on death during attempts at police restraint reveals that autopsy-negative deaths continue to occur regardless of the type of restraint used; the deaths are unexplained by gross anatomic or microscopic autopsy findings, toxicology testing, scene investigation, or medical history. Nontraumatic deaths of agitated individuals during or shortly after lateral vascular neck restraint, the hogtie restraint, four-point restraint, and now even taser restraints continue to occur. When these deaths cannot be adequately explained by injuries produced or lethal pathophysiology of the procedures themselves, it is clear that the deaths are coincident with but not caused by the restraint procedure. Deaths in such circumstances can be reasonably attributed to sudden death precipitated by acute stress response.

Numerous events that have been described by participants in and witnesses to unexpected deaths during police restraint procedures can be explained by and are consistent with the pathophysiology of the acute stress response *(65–69)* (Table 3). The timing of sudden death is consistent with the time course of the acute stress response cascade. The epinephrine pools released from the chromaffin adrenomedullary cells occur rapidly, and, in some, may be followed by a delayed or "depo-effect" of epinephrine. A common observation recorded by police is the sudden unresponsiveness of the detainee, which progresses to cardiopulmonary arrest after the struggle has ceased. The characteristic of the epinephrine release may account for sudden collapse both during restraint or immediately after restraint procedures have been applied. During police confrontation, the anticipatory component of stress may intensify the physiological stress response and make the individual more susceptible to a sudden unexpected death during the ensuing physical component of restraint. Furthermore, police frequently report that the struggling detainee appeared unfazed by pain or pepper spray and could successfully resist the physical efforts of multiple law enforcement personnel. This is consistent with the analgesia and enhanced physical strength produced by the acute stress response. Unexpected deaths during restraint are more likely to occur when the victim has ingested drugs that can potentiate the neuroendocrine catecholamine response such as amphetamines or cocaine. Finally, lactic acidosis has been recently reported in several cases of

### Table 3
### Similarities Between the Effects of the Acute Stress Response and Reports
### of Sudden Unexpected Death During Police Restraint

| Characteristics of death during police restraint | Characteristics of acute stress response |
|---|---|
| • Increased muscle strength | • Epinephrine causes increased blood flow to active skeletal muscles |
| • Decreased pain perception | • β-endorphin is released from pituitary |
| • Unresponsiveness noted during or just after restraint is accomplished | • Rapid release pool of epinephrine from adrenal chromaffin cell |
| | • Depo-effect of epinephrine actions |
| • Unexplained cardiorespiratory arrest | • Epinephrine can produce fatal cardiac arrhythmias and pulmonary edema |
| • No anatomic cause of death identified | • Neuroendocrine cascade is a functional response, not a structural change |
| • Lactic acidosis reported | • Lactic acidosis results from increased basal metabolic rate |
| • Psychotic and/or drug induced abnormal behavior noted | • Individual's perception of the event determines the response |

autopsy-negative restraint deaths, a finding that can be explained by the effects of epinephrine released as a result of the acute stress response *(39,45,46)*.

The task of the pathologist investigating sudden death during restraint is to develop a method of analytical thinking in order to reason about causality. In epidemiological terms, a cause is an act, event, or state that initiates or permits, alone or in conjunction with other causes, a sequence of events resulting in the effect *(70)*. It is helpful to think about sudden death during custody or restraint in this context, examining the contributions of disease and injury (structural) and acute stress physiology (functional) to the death (Fig. 2). Each of these three areas should be evaluated to determine whether each item is present and sufficient, alone or in combination, to cause death.

When disease and injury from restraint alone are inadequate to explain death, the only process remaining to consider is an adverse physiological outcome of the neuroendocrine cascade triggered by the acute stress response to restraint. The diagnosis of death owing to the acute stress response during restraint can be the conclusion only after a rigorous scene investigation with reconstruction of the events from witness statements, police reports, and medical

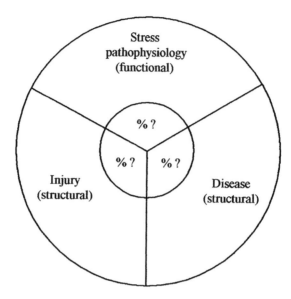

**Fig. 2.** Evaluation of cause of death during restraint based on complete medico-legal death investigation. Cause means present and sufficient, alone or in combination, to account for death.

records from emergency responders. The autopsy must be thorough with complete histology, electrolytes, and toxicology. Previous medical records should be examined, if available.

## CONCLUSION

The occurrence of death as a result of the acute stress response is a rare, but real phenomenon. The acute stress response includes adaptive measures to prepare the animal for fight or escape. The neuroendocrine cascade precipitated by this response allows for complex types of responses in many different organs. The response is influenced by the way the individual perceives the event, psychological factors based on the individual, and any underlying diseases or drugs present. Sudden death from the acute stress response can occur unpredictably and has been associated with physical restraint. The forensic pathologist should expect to see sudden death without significant structural changes at autopsy.

## ACKNOWLEDGMENTS

The author gratefully acknowledges Angel Desmarais for her expert preparation of the manuscript; Colin Murphy of Murphy and Murphy, Providence, RI for Fig. 1 graphics and Joseph R. Winn, Jr. for his editorial skills.

# REFERENCES

1. Cannon WB. Voices from the past "voodoo" death. Am J Health 2002;92: 1593–1596.
2. Von Euler US. Epinephrine and norepinephrine adrenaline and nor adrenaline distribution and action. Pharmacol Rev 1954;6:15–22.
3. Cannon BC. Voodoo death. American Anthropologist 1942;44:169–181.
4. Brown W. New Zealand and Its Aborigines: Being an Account of the Aborigines, Trade and Resources of the Colony; and the Advantages It Now Presents as a Field for Emigration and the Investment of Capital. Smith, Elder, London, 1845.
5. Selye H. The physiology and pathology of exposure to stress. In: A Treatise Based on the Concepts of the General Adaptation Syndrome and the Diseases of Adaptation. Acta Inc. Montreal, 1950.
6. Selye H. A syndrome produced by diverse noxious agents. Nature Lond 1936;138:32.
7. Pacak K, Palkovits M. Stressor specificity of central neuroendocrine responses: implications for stress-related disorders. Endocrine Rev 2001;22(4):502–548.
8. Holmes TH, Rahe RH. Journal of Psychosomatic research. 1967;11:213–218.
9. Lazarus RS, Folkman S. Stress Appraisal and Coping. Springer-Verlag, New York, 1984.
10. Tomaka J, Blascovich J, Kibler J, Ernst J. Cognitive and physiological antecedents of threat and challenge appraisal. J Pers Soc Psychol 1997;73:63–72.
11. Axelrod J, Reisine TD. Stress hormones: their interaction and regulation. Science 1984;224:452–459.
12. O'Connor TM, O'Halloran DJ, Shanahan R. The stress response and the hypothalamic–pituitary–adrenal axis: From molecule to melancholia. QJ Med 2000;93:323–333.
13. Aunis D, Langley K. Physiological aspects of exocytosis in chromaffin cells of the adrenal medulla. Acta Psysiol Scanda 1999;167:89–97.
14. Esler M, Jennings G, Lambert G, et al. Overflow of catecholamine neurotransmitters to the circulation: source, fate, and functions. Physiol Rev 1990;70:963–985.
15. Richter SD, Schwimeyer TH, Schedlowski M, et al. Time kinetics of the endocrine response to acute psychological stress. J Clin Endocrinol Metab 1996;81:1956–1960.
16. Amit Z, Galina ZH. Stress-induced analgesia: adaptive pain suppression. Physiol Rev 2000;66:1091–120.
17. Clutter WE, Bier DM, Shah SD, et al. Epinephrine plasma metabolic clearance rates and physiologic thresholds for metabolic and hemodynamic actions in man. J Clin Invest 1980;66:94–101.
18. Stratton JR, Pfeiffer MA, Ritchie JL, et al. Hemodynamic effects of epinephrine: concentration-effect study in humans. J Appl Physiol 1985;58:1199–206.
19. Tang W. Use of epinephrine as vasopressor agent during cardiopulmonary resuscitation another example of a double edged sword. Crit Care Med 2000;122:1671–1672.
20. Bahr R, Hostmark AT, Newsholme EA, et al. Effect of exercise on recovery changes in plasma levels of FFA, glycerol, glucose and catecholamines. Acta Physiol Scand 1991;143:105–115.

21. Aguilera G. Corticotropin releasing hormone. Receptor regulation and the stress response. TEM 1998;9:329–336.

22. Halasz B. The hypothalamus as an endocrine organ: The science of neuroendoendocrinology. In: Conn, PM, Freeman ME eds., Neuroendocrinology in Physiology and Medicine. Humana Press, Totowa NJ, 2000, pp 3–21.

23. Hargreaves KM, Muller GP, Dubner R, et al. Corticotropin-releasing releasing factor (CRF) produces analgesia in humans and rats. Brain Res 1987;422:154–157.

24. Miller DB, O'Callaghan JP. Neuroendocrine aspects of the response to stress. Metabolism 2002;51:5–10.

25. Selye H. Thymus and adrenals in the response of the organism to injuries and intoxications. Br J Exp Pathol 1936;17:234–248.

26. Kubo T, Okatani H, Nishigori Y, Hagiwara Y, Fukumori R, Goshima Y. Involvement of the medial amygdaloid nucleus in restraint stress-induced pressor responses in rats. Neuroscience Letters 2004;354:84–86.

27. Palkovits M, Baffi JS, Pacak K. Stress-induces Fos-like immunoreactivity in the pons and the medulla oblongata of rats. Stress 1997;1:155–168.

28. Palkovits M, Baffi JS, Dvori S. Neuronal organization of stress response. Pain-induced c-fos expression in brain stem catecholaminergic cell groups. Ann NY Acad Sci 1995;771:313–326.

29. Pacak K, Palkovits M, Makino S, Kopin IJ, Goldstein JS. Brainstem hemisection decreases corticotropin-releasing hormone mRNA in the paraventricular nucleus but not in the central amygdaloid nucleus. J Neuroendocrinol 1996;8:543–551.

30. Bartanusz V, Jezova D, Bertini LT, Tilders FJ, Aubry JM, Kiss JZ. Stress-induced increase in vasopressin and corticotropin-releasing factor expression in hypophysiotrophic paraventricular neurons. Endocrinology 1993;132:895–902.

31. Cahill AL, Eertmoed AL, Mangoura D, et al. Differential regulation of phenylethanolamine N-methyltransferase expression in two distinct subpopulations in bovine chromaffin cells. J Neurochem 1996;67:1217–1224.

32. Wurtman RJ. Stress and the adrenocortical control of epinephrine synthesis. Metabolism 2002;51:11–14.

33. Kaada B. The sudden infant death syndrome induced by "the fear paralysis reflex"? Medical Hypothesis 1987;22:347–356.

34. Scavo D, Bartletta C, Vagiri D, Letizia C. Adrenocorticotropic hormone, beta-endorphin, cortisol, growth hormone and prolactin circulating levels in nineteen athletes before and after half-marathon. J Sport Med Phys Fitness 1991;31:401–406.

35. McEwen BS. Protective and damaging effects of stress mediators. Seminars in Medicine of the Beth Israel Deaconess Medical Center 1998;338:171–179.

36. Verrier RL, Mittleman MA. Life-threatening cardiovascular consequences of anger in patients with coronary heart disease. Cardiol Clin 1996;14:289–307.

37. Reich P, DeSilva RA, Lown B, et al. Acute psychological disturbances preceding life-threatening ventricular arrhythmias. JAMA 1981;246:233–235.

38. Herd JA. Cardiovascular response to stress. The American Physiological Society 1991;71:305–330.

39. Kurachek SC., Rockoff MA. Inadvertent intravenous admission of racemic epinephrine. JAMA 1985;253:1441–1442.
40. Lepeschkin E, Marchet H, Schroeder G, et al. Effects of epinephrine and norepinephrine on the electrocardiogram of 100 normal subjects. Am J Cardiol 1960;5:594–603.
41. Mazzeo RS, Bender PR, Brooks GA, et al. Arterial catecholamine responses during exercise with acute and chronic high-altitude exposure. Am J Physiol 1991;261:E419–E424.
42. Serda SM, Wei ET. Epinephrine-induced pulmonary edema in rats is inhibited by corticotropin-releasing factor. Pharmacol Res 1992;26:85–91.
43. Ganeshan N, Bihari D. Life-threatening hyperkalaemia after cardiac surgery. Lancet 1996;348:755.
44. Kolendorf K, Moller BB. Lactic acidosis in epinephrine poisoning. Acta Med Scand 1974;196:465–466.
45. Hick JL, Smith SW, Lynch MT. Metabolic acidosis in restraint-associated cardiac arrest: a case series. Acad Emerg Med 1999;6:239–243.
46. Chan TC, Neuman T, et al. Metabolic acidosis in restraint-associated cardiac arrest (correspondence). Acad Emerg Med 1999;6:1075–1077.
47. Laposata EA. Cocaine-induced heart disease: mechanisms and pathology. J Thorac Imaging 1991;6(1):68–75.
48. Wetli CV, Fishbain DA. Cocaine-induced psychosis and sudden death in recreational cocaine users. J Forensic Sci 1985;30:873–880.
49. Ruttenbir AJ, Lawler-Heavner J, Yin M, et al. Fatal excited delirium following cocaine use: epidemiologic findings provide new evidence for mechanisms of cocaine toxicity. J Forensic Sci 1997;42(1):25–31.
50. Laposata EL, Hale P, Polkis A. Evaluation of sudden death in psychiatric patients with special reference to phenothiazine therapy: forensic pathology. J Forensic Sci 1988;33(2):432–440.
51. Wendkos MH. Acute exhaustive mania in sudden death and psychiatric illness. Spectrum Publications, New York, 1978, pp. 165–177.
52. Servoss SJ, Januzzi JL, Muller JE. Triggers of acute coronary syndromes. Prog Cardiovasc Dis 2002;44:369–380.
53. McMurtry JP, Wexler BC. Hypersensitivity of spontaneously hypersensitive rats (SHR) to heat, ether, and immobilization. Endocrinology 1981;108:1730–1735.
54. Tan HL, Hou CJY, Lauer MR, et al. Electrophysiologic mechanisms of the long QT interval syndromes and torsades de pointes. Ann Intern Med 1995;122: 701–714.
55. Towbin JA, Vatta M. Molecular biology and the prolonged QT syndromes. Am J Med 2001;110:385–398.
56. Liu BA, Juurlink DN. Drugs and the QT interval-caveat doctor. N Engl J Med 2004;351(11):1053–1056.
57. Straus SM, Bleumink GS, Dieleman JP, et al. Antipsychotics and the risk of sudden cardiac death. Arch Intern Med 2004;164:1293–1297.
58. McEwen BS. Protective and damaging effects of stress mediators: The good and bad sides of the response to stress. Metabolism 2002;51:2–4.

59. Hamet P, Tremblay J. Genetic determinants of the stress response in cardiovascular disease. Metabolism 2002;51:15–24.
60. Dishy V, Sofowora GG, Xie HG, et al. The effect of common polymorphisms of the β2-adrenergic receptor on agonist-medicated vascular desensitization. N Engl J Med 2001;345:1030–1035.
61. Johansson SR, Ake H. Age and sex differences in cardiovascular reactivity to adrenergic agonists, mental stress and isometric exercise in normal subjects. Scand J Clin Lab Invest 1988;48:183–191.
62. Blumenthal JA, Emery MA, Walsh MA, et al. Exercise training in healthy type A middle-aged men: effects on behavioral and cardiovascular responses. Psychosom Med 1988;50:418–433.
63. Robinson BE. Death by destruction of will. Arch Intern Med 1995;155:2250–2251.
64. Robinson BE, Sucholeiki R, Schocken D. Sudden death and resisted mechanical restraint: a case report. J Am Geriatr Soc 1993;41:424–425.
65. Pollanen MS, Chiasson DA, Cairns JT, Young JG. Unexpected death related to restraint for excited delirium: a retrospective study of deaths in police custody and in the community. CMAJ 1998;158:1603–1607.
66. Pestaner JP, Southall PE. Sudden death during arrest and phencyclidine intoxication. Am J Forensic Med Pathol 2003;24:119–122.
67. O'Halloran RL, Frank JG. Asphyxial death during prone restraint revisited. Am J Forensic Med Pathol 2000;21(1):39–52.
68. Reay DT, Flinger CL, Stilwell AD, Arnold J. Positional asphyxia during law enforcement transport. Am J Forensic Med Pathol 1992;13(2):90–97.
69. Berenson A. As police use of tasers soars, questions over safety emerge. The New York Times 2004;CLIII(52,914).
70. Hill AB. The environment and disease: association or causation? In: Greenland S, ed., Evolution of Epidemiologic Ideas: Annotated Readings on Concepts in Methods. Epidemiology Resources Inc., MA, 1987, pp. 7–12.

# Chapter 6

# The Role of Illicit Drug Use in Sudden In-Custody Death

*Aaron B. Schneir and Richard F. Clark*

## INTRODUCTION

A substantial portion of all the deaths reviewed by medical examiners and coroners relates to the use of cocaine and other illicit drugs *(1)*. Not surprisingly, because of the illegality of these substances, many of these individuals die while in the custody of law enforcement. In fact, forensic pathologists have often divided these drug-related custody deaths into four different categories: (a) death during arrest and transport or soon thereafter; (b) death within 12 hours of arrest: (c) death after 12 hours, but within a few days to weeks; and (d) death after days to weeks of incarceration *(2)*. Death within 12 hours of arrest is commonly associated with massive drug overdose, such as can occur with smugglers who conceal drugs within body cavities, an act that is known as "body packing." Deaths that occur days to weeks or longer after incarceration can be associated with drug withdrawal or other natural causes related to drug use *(2)*.

This chapter focuses on the category of drug-related custody deaths that occur during the time of the initial law enforcement encounter, arrest, and transport of the individual, or soon thereafter. These deaths have common features in terms of the presentation of the individual and the sudden, unexpected nature of the individual's demise, such that the term *sudden in-custody death syndrome* has been applied to these deaths. A clear association exists between illicit drug

From: *Forensic Science and Medicine: Sudden Deaths in Custody*
Edited by: D. L. Ross and T. C. Chan © Humana Press Inc., Totowa, NJ

use and this syndrome. This chapter elaborates on the contribution of illicit drug use to the sudden in-custody death syndrome.

## DRUGS INVOLVED IN SUDDEN IN-CUSTODY DEATH SYNDROME

The association between sudden in-custody death syndrome and illicit drug use seemed clear from some of the first case reports of these deaths in the medical literature *(3)*. Drug use in these individuals is often detailed by a history of exposure to an agent, characteristic physical findings of drug intoxication, and confirmatory laboratory testing. The illicit drugs most frequently associated are all sympathomimetic agents and include cocaine, methamphetamine, phencyclidine (PCP), and lysergic acid (LSD) *(4–12)*.

An article published in 1985 entitled "Cocaine-Induced Psychosis and Sudden Death in Recreational Cocaine Users" by Wetli and Fishbain first documented an association of cocaine intoxication and sudden death *(3)*. In their series, five of the seven individuals were in police custody at the time of death. Subsequently, multiple series and case reports have consistently documented an association between the use of certain illicit drugs and sudden in-custody death, often associated with restraint *(4,6–16)*. In one retrospective case series of 18 cases of sudden restraint deaths, 78% had the presence of a stimulant drug (cocaine, amphetamine, or PCP) and 45% had known chronic cocaine use *(4)*.

Cocaine use was found to be present in the majority of cases in an extensive review of the literature examining the factors associated with sudden in-custody death *(6)*. Second to cocaine is the increasingly popular methamphetamine. Far fewer cases are reported with PCP and even fewer with LSD. Not infrequently, more than one illicit drug is detected in an individual who suffers sudden in-custody death. In Stratton's series, some individuals had the presence of both cocaine and amphetamine, and one had the presence of both an amphetamine and PCP *(4)*. The significance of detecting more than one illicit drug in the setting of sudden in-custody death is not clear. It may reflect intentional polysubstance use or merely use of adulterated specimens. Other drugs, including ethanol, marijuana, and therapeutic agents are occasionally detected, usually in addition to the illicit sympathomimetic agents classically associated with the syndrome.

Of particular interest may be the combination of cocaine use with ethanol. Concurrent use of both agents leads to the formation of a hepatically derived metabolite, cocaethylene. Cocaethylene has pharmacological properties similar to that of cocaine, but has a plasma half-life that is three to five times longer *(17)*. In a mouse model, cocaethylene was more potent in mediating lethality than cocaine *(18)*. Cocaethylene levels have been documented in those suffering sudden in-custody death *(5,12)*. In Ross' series, the most common mixture of drugs was cocaine and ethanol *(6)*.

The particular danger of cocaine use may be reflected in the fact that cocaine is the most common drug used by those who have died from sudden in-custody death syndrome. In a rat model, it has been shown that restraint stress following cocaine administration increases mortality *(19)*. However, the particular distribution of drugs associated with these deaths may also at least partially reflect changing drug-use patterns.

## Pattern of Drug Use in Sudden In-Custody Death

Sudden in-custody deaths associated with illicit drug use are not simply the result of an overdose of the offending drug. Clearly, all of the drugs associated with this syndrome, when used in great excess or "overdose," can cause death in the absence of any extenuating circumstances. Forensic drug testing, an essential aspect of any custody death investigation, may be helpful in distinguishing between these two entities, and has provided some insights into the pattern of drug use in those suffering from sudden death.

It must be recognized, however, that particularly with cocaine, there is a wide range of drug levels at which individuals develop symptoms of toxicity *(20)*. In fact no scientific association exists for the designation of lethal and nonlethal blood cocaine levels *(2,21)*. Blaho et al, in an emergency department population found no statistical correlation between cocaine or any metabolite concentrations and the severity of clinical symptoms, disposition, need for treatment, or outcome *(20)*. Such data suggest to some that a critical element in certain manifestations of toxicity, such as the state of excited delirium, is chronic use of cocaine *(22)*. It has been postulated that chronic cocaine use may lead to critical anatomic and neurochemical adaptations that may predispose individuals to such conditions as excited delirium and death.

Multiple series have documented that the amount of cocaine measured in those suffering from sudden in-custody death is similar to other recreational users, and lower than those associated with overdose *(3,14)*. Pollanen et al. reported postmortem cocaine and benzoylecgonine (a primary metabolite of cocaine and what most qualitative screens actually detect) levels when present in a series of individuals who died from sudden in-custody death syndrome, and compared them to two control groups: (a) recreational cocaine users who died of an etiology clearly separate from cocaine use, and (b) individuals whose deaths were attributed to cocaine intoxication itself. Although statistics are not reported to determine significance, it was found that the mean serum cocaine concentration in the in-custody deaths was similar to that of recreational users but much lower than that of people whose deaths were attributed to pure cocaine intoxication. Furthermore, benzoylecgonine serum concentrations were higher in the individuals suffering sudden in-custody death than in the recreational users, but lower than those deaths attributed to pure cocaine intoxication.

Multiple interpretations of this data are possible. It seems clear that those suffering from sudden in-custody death had not simply "overdosed" on cocaine. Also, the concentration of cocaine found associated with recreational use may in fact be sufficient to induce a state of excited delirium. Finally, because benzoylecgonine has a much longer half-life than the parent cocaine compound, the higher level of benzoylecgonine in the excited delirium individuals suggests repeated recent use or "binging."

Although this article provides insight into the pattern of cocaine use in the patients that they studied, simply not enough research has addressed this topic to make conclusive statements regarding the typical pattern of cocaine use in those who suffer sudden in-custody death. Additionally, much less information exists regarding the pattern of drug use with the other drugs associated.

## SIMILARITY IN DRUGS ASSOCIATED WITH SUDDEN IN-CUSTODY DEATH

All of the illicit drugs associated with the sudden in-custody death syndrome are considered sympathomimetic agents. That is, they are capable of inducing a state of sympathetic dominance (fight or flight). Cocaine and methamphetamine act to increase dopamine in the central nervous system, and norepinephrine peripherally. Cocaine does so by reuptake inhibition and methamphetamine by release of the transmitters. The resulting excess, centrally of dopamine, and peripherally of norepinephrine helps explain much of both the desired and adverse effects of these agents. Dopamine excess centrally is implicated in the desired euphoria, but also in addiction, agitation, psychosis, and hyperthermia. Norepinephrine excess peripherally induces characteristic signs of intoxication, which include mydriasis (dilated pupils), diaphoresis, tachycardia, and hypertension. The vasoconstrictive properties of norepinephrine excess explain many of the associated complications. PCP and LSD act via different mechanisms but are capable of inducing a similar sympathetic dominance state. PCP acts through various receptors including the methyl-D-aspartate receptor to induce its effects, whereas LSD acts through serotonergic receptors.

## THE CONTRIBUTION OF ILLICIT DRUG USE TO SUDDEN IN-CUSTODY DEATH

Despite a clear temporal association of sudden in-custody death syndrome and use of certain illicit drugs, defining their exact contribution to death has proved quite difficult. Multiple reasons account for this. To begin with, as described elsewhere in this volume, the deaths themselves are characterized by the absence of a clearly identifiable etiology. Illicit drug use is just one of many conditions that has been associated with these deaths, which likely are multifactorial. In addition, relatively little medical literature exists on the topic. The information in this chapter derives from what is published primarily in retrospective reviews, case series, and case reports, of individuals who suffered from sudden in-custody death. In these reports, physical examination findings, cardiac monitoring, laboratory testing, and other aspects are not always rigorously documented. Animal models have been used to help elucidate the mechanisms responsible for sudden deaths. Although some are extremely helpful in evaluating certain mechanisms, all are limited, most notably by potential interspecies differences.

The understandable lack of prospective studies on this topic makes it difficult to ascertain definitively how frequently these types of death occur. How often individuals are in apparently identical situations that seem to predispose to sudden death, yet suffer no adverse sequelae is unknown. It also must be emphasized that although an association clearly exists between sudden in-custody deaths and recent illicit drug use, the association is not universal. Nearly identical types of deaths have occurred in the absence of recent drug use *(14)*. Finally, the detection of an illicit drug on toxicological tests by no means necessarily means that it was contributory to the death, but simply that is was detected.

## POTENTIAL MECHANISMS FOR THE ROLE OF ILLICIT DRUG USE IN SUDDEN IN-CUSTODY DEATH

Despite the many limitations that make it difficult to elucidate the contribution of illicit drug use to sudden death, the association is a strong one. Additionally, the association is with a particular class of agents, namely the sympathomimetics, suggesting common mechanisms by which these drugs may contribute to death. The following discussion elaborates on some of these mechanisms, which include excited delirium, cardiac dysfunction, metabolic acidosis, hyperthermia, convulsions, hyperkalemia, and respiratory dysfunction.

## Excited Delirium

Characteristic behavior, referred to as agitated or excited delirium, is one of the hallmarks found in those who suffer from sudden in-custody death. In fact, it is the behavior itself that often initiates law enforcement contact. These individuals, whether under the influence of an illicit agent or not, manifest paranoia, hyperactivity, psychosis, violence, and even when maximally restrained, continue to struggle. Use of all of the illicit sympathomimetic agents may precipitate such behavior, which by itself may be highly dangerous. Furthermore, it is thought that chronic use of certain agents, particularly cocaine, may predispose individuals to developing excited delirium, even in the absence of acute intoxication.

Paradoxically, analysis of those individuals who suffer sudden in-custody death despite not having used illicit drugs may actually provide insight into the contribution illicit drug use has to these deaths. Multiple series document the absence of illicit drug use in a percentage of those who suffer sudden in-custody death *(4,8,12,14)*. In one series, 12 of 21 individuals (57%) were found to be suffering from a psychiatric disorder and not under the influence of illicit drugs *(14)*. Individuals who suffer sudden in-custody death in the absence of illicit drug use are almost universally experiencing psychosis and often suffer from psychiatric conditions such as schizophrenia or bipolar disorder. These individuals actually appear intoxicated, and clinically may be impossible to distinguish from those in whom a sympathomimetic drug was the precipitant.

Despite different etiologies, the resulting outward clinical appearance is nearly identical, suggesting the presence of similar internal pathophysiology. Such pathophysiology is undoubtedly marked by catecholamine excess, a proposed mechanism of sudden death from various causes (*see* the following discussion on cardiac dysfunction). Therefore, one major contribution that illicit sympathomimetic agents have to these deaths is the precipitation of excited delirium itself, a pathophysiological state, regardless of etiology, that is a risk factor for death. As discussed here, some of the drugs may have additional mechanisms that further contribute to the risk of death.

## Cardiac Dysfunction

Rapid cardiac dysfunction is a potential mechanism by which illicit drug use may contribute to sudden death. Such a mechanism, which could manifest as a lethal dysrhythmia, would help explain the abrupt nature of these deaths, and the characteristic lack of identifiable etiology found at autopsy. Although no universal dysrhythmia has been reported in those individuals who had cardiac monitoring at the time of decompensation, the mechanism itself seems plausible. A common pathophysiological state of catecholamine excess, that all of the sympathomimetic agents can induce, could be responsible. The additional particularly adverse cardiac effects of cocaine, could help explain why it is the drug most associated with these deaths.

Catecholamine excess may be a crucial common mechanism of sudden cardiac death in various situations *(23)*. Intense emotional stress precipitating an acute transient cardiomyopathy has been documented in humans and has recently been shown to be associated with catecholamine excess *(24,25)*. Catecholamine excess is associated with a unique type of myocyte injury referred to as contraction-band necrosis seen only in histologically prepared cardiac tissue (would not be seen on a routine autopsy). Such injury has been documented in clinical states of catecholamine excess such as pheochromocytoma, and subarachnoid hemorrhage *(26,27)*. It has also been observed postmortem in individuals who die under terrifying circumstances such as asthma and violent assault *(28,29)*.

Not surprisingly, in one study of cocaine-associated deaths, a 93% incidence of contraction band necrosis in the myocardium was found *(30)*. However, of individuals suffering sudden in-custody death who have had histological specimens described, these characteristic findings have typically not been found. Wetli and Fishbain detailed that cardiac abnormalities on microscopic analysis were specifically excluded in six cases *(3)*. In O'Halloran's series of 21 cases, many individuals were documented to have microscopically normal cardiac tissue *(12)*.

The combination of catecholamine excess and cocaine intoxication may be particularly dangerous, and may help explain why it is the drug most associated with these deaths. In a rat model of cocaine poisoning attempting to emulate a "stress state" by infusing intravenous catecholamines, it was found that elevated catecholamines enhanced the circulatory toxicity of cocaine. Interestingly, in this model, the interaction seemed to occur by a pharmocokinetic interaction in which catecholamine administration appeared to elevate serum cocaine levels *(31)*.

Cocaine has well-known adverse cardiac effects. Induction of cardiac ischemia is a potentially significant method that cocaine use may contribute to cardiac dysfunction. Cocaine use not only increases myocardial oxygen demand by causing hypertension and tachycardia, but also decreases myocardial oxygen supply by causing vasoconstriction of coronary arteries and small intramyocardial vessels *(32,33)*. This vasoconstriction is more pronounced at sites of atherosclerosis *(34)*. It is likely that methamphetamine has similar effects. This adverse combination may be particularly harmful in the setting of extreme myocardial oxygen demand, as would undoubtedly be the case in individuals maximally exerting themselves. It may explain why even minimal atherosclerotic lesions, not deemed at autopsy to be significant, may actually be functionally quite so, in the presence of cocaine use. Cocaine use itself is actually a risk factor for the development of such atherosclerotic lesions *(35)*.

Chronic use of cocaine and methamphetamine is also associated with the development of cardiomyopathy, a condition that predisposes to dysrhythmias *(36,37)*. The percentage of individuals who suffer sudden in-custody death who have any degree of such cardiomyopathy is unclear. However, at least in one series of deaths from this syndrome, nearly half were chronic cocaine users *(4)*. Both cocaine and the metabolite it forms with ethanol, cocaethylene, have sodium channel-blocking properties *(38,39)*. This property is associated with myocardial conduction impairment, cardiac dysrhythmias, and in massive overdose is likely a major factor in mediating death *(40)*. With recreational use patterns typical of those who die under restraint, it remains unclear exactly what contribution sodium channel blockade has to cocaine-related sudden death. It has been suggested that it is significant, but only in combination with ischemia, sympathetic excess, and structural heart disease *(41)*. The long half-life of cocaethylene may prolong the period in which such an adverse combination could occur.

## Metabolic Acidosis

The presence of a severe metabolic acidosis may be a major contributing factor in the etiology of sudden in-custody deaths. Profound metabolic acidosis itself, regardless of etiology, may lead to cardiovascular instability and collapse. Severe acidosis has been described in those suffering from sudden in-custody death associated with illicit drug use *(15,16)*. Hick et al. reported a series of five individuals who had used cocaine and in classic sudden restraint-type situations suffered cardiopulmonary arrest with profound metabolic acidosis *(15)*. They felt the extreme acidemia documented in their series was far beyond what is typically found in sudden deaths in other situations, and they postulated that it might have been a significant contributing factor to these deaths.

Strenuous exertion alone is associated with a lactic acidosis *(42,43)*. Additionally, it is likely that the state of excited delirium allows for exertion far beyond normal physiological limits. Furthermore, the presence of a sympathomimetic agent may exacerbate this acidosis. A rat model has demonstrated that when exercise is performed after cocaine administration, the combined effect on lactic acidosis is synergistic *(44)*. This exaggerated response has been documented in humans as well *(45)*. Such acidosis has also been shown in vitro to worsen the sodium channel-mediated cardiac conduction associated with cocaine *(46)*.

It remains unclear exactly how sympathomimetic agents exacerbate acidosis. By inhibiting mitochondrial function, cocaine may cause exercising muscle to rely more on anaerobic adenosine triphosphate production with a corresponding accumulation of lactic acid *(47)*. It has been postulated that, by causing peripheral vasoconstriction, sympathomimetic drugs may impede clearance of generated lactate. However, at least in a rat model, it has been demonstrated that chemical antagonism to peripheral vasoconstriction does not affect the degree of lactic acidosis *(44)*. Although the exact role that significant acidosis plays in sudden in-custody death is unclear, it is likely that sympathomimetic agents may contribute to it.

## Hyperthermia

Hyperthermia, defined as elevation of core body temperature secondary to thermoregulatory failure, is common in those suffering sudden in-custody death, and is likely to be at least contributory, if not crucial to why these individuals die. It is again by no coincidence that by various mechanisms, all of the illicit drugs associated with sudden restraint may produce hyperthermia *(48–51)*.

Some degree of hyperthermia is likely present in the vast majority, if not all, of those with sudden in-custody death. In one retrospective series of excited delirium deaths that also included nonrestrained individuals, 97% were found to be hyperthermic *(9)*. In a retrospective review of 61 sudden restraint deaths, rectal temperature measurement at some point was available in 42. The mean was found to be 104°F with a range of 100–108°F *(6)*. In their initial documentation of sudden in-custody death, Wetli and Fishbain consistently documented significantly elevated postmortem temperatures. One individual had a rectal temperature of 41°C (106°F) almost 2 hours after death. Occasionally, normal postmortem temperatures are documented, which certainly does not exclude the possibility of hyperthermia at the time of death *(12)*.

The mechanism by which sympathomimetic agents contribute to hyperthermia is likely multifactorial. Extreme exertion alone, even in the absence of illicit drug use may lead to severe hyperthermia. This is the classic pattern of exertional heat stroke seen most commonly in unconditioned athletes and military recruits. By inducing the behavior of excited delirium, all of the illicit sympathomimetic agents may similarly contribute to hyperthermia by this exertional mechanism in which a significant amount of heat is generated. Furthermore, drug-induced excited delirium can preclude normal behavior measures of limiting further muscular movement that would otherwise help in lowering their temperature.

Additionally, cocaine and methamphetamine may also induce hyperthermia directly by activating particular dopamine receptors in the central nervous system *(52,53)*. The mechanism by which LSD does so is likely via interaction with serotonergic receptors. This direct effect explains why sympathomimetic-induced hyperthermia may occur independent of increased motor activity, as is seen in certain animal models and clinical situations *(52)*. Finally, the resulting catecholamine excess induced by sympathomimetic agents leads peripherally to vasoconstriction, effectively limiting heat dissipation that could otherwise occur via the skin surface.

The contribution of climate in the setting of sudden in-custody death is usually not addressed in the literature. If climate were indeed important, it would likely be related to hyperthermia, particularly in the setting of intoxication with certain agents. One series found that excited delirium deaths (included nonrestraint deaths) occurred more often in the summer than in any other season *(9)*. Any ambient environmental temperature elevation or increased humidity will limit heat-releasing mechanisms and likely exacerbate any hyperthermia experienced in the setting of sudden in-custody death. Furthermore, in a rat model, the ability of cocaine to induce hyperthermia correlates with ambient temperature elevation *(54)*. This may help explain why the risk of death associated with cocaine has been shown to further increase during hot weather *(55)*. Heat-response mechanisms may be altered in users of certain drugs. Varied endocrinological responses to heat in those addicted to cocaine have been demonstrated *(56)*.

Intoxication from illicit sympathomimetic agents undoubtedly contributes to the hyperthermia observed in those who suffer a sudden in-custody death. Regardless of the mechanisms responsible, severe hyperthermia itself is life-threatening and at minimum is likely contributory to why deaths occur in these settings.

## Convulsions

Convulsions may occur as manifestations of toxicity with cocaine and methamphetamine *(57)*. Regardless of etiology, convulsions themselves can be associated with various complications including metabolic acidosis and hyperthermia, which would exacerbate pre-existing pathophysiological states in those under restraint with excited delirium.

Convulsions, however, are clearly not a universal occurrence in those who die from sudden in-custody death syndrome. With regards to cocaine, this is actually not unexpected, as convulsions are one of the few dose-related effects of cocaine and are more typical of actual overdose than recreational use *(58)*. In much of the literature, in fact, convulsions are not described. Two retrospective series are notable exceptions. In a series by Ruttenber et al. that reviewed fatal excited delirium cases that were not necessarily under restraint, 27% were recorded as having had a convulsion *(9)*. Similarly, in a series by Ross of 61 sudden restraint deaths, "seizures or uncontrolled shaking were observed in 54% of the victims" *(6)*. Although these series do not delineate which individuals suffering a convulsion were under the influence of a drug, it seems likely that many were. Documentation of status epilepticus, a condition defined by either repetitive or persistent convulsions, which is associated with significant mortality has not been described in the setting of sudden in-custody death syndrome. In those instances in which a convulsion occurs, the convulsion itself must be considered a potential contributing factor to death.

## Hyperkalemia

Hyperkalemia (elevation of blood potassium), is an appealing mechanism by which the sympathomimetic agents may contribute to sudden in-custody death syndrome. Hyperkalemia, regardless of etiology, can lead to fatal dysrhythmias, a mechanism as discussed previously that would help explain the abruptness of these deaths and lack of anatomical etiology found at autopsy. However, at least from the limited information we have on these deaths, such a mechanism seems unlikely.

Sympathomimetic drug-associated hyperkalemia results mostly from rhabdomyolysis, defined as skeletal muscle breakdown. Rhabdomyolysis is clearly associated with both extreme exertion and poisoning with all of the illicit drugs associated with sudden in-custody death syndrome *(59,60)*. With sympathomimetic agents, it is likely that the combination of extreme exertion and hyperthermia, coupled to peripheral vascular constriction, may lead to muscle ischemia and ultimately cell death. Cells may then release stored potassium, and components of muscle may cause renal damage that can diminish the ability to excrete potassium. Additionally, metabolic acidosis leads to transcellular shifting of potassium into blood, further increasing serum levels.

Significant hyperkalemia seems plausible in the setting of sudden death conditions in which extreme exertion is occurring in the setting of sympathomimetic drug intoxication and severe metabolic acidosis. However, although pulseless electrical activity rhythms have been described with sudden in-custody deaths, characteristic life-threatening sinusoidal rhythms of hyperkalemia have not been detailed. Furthermore, the few potassium levels reported in those suffering from sudden in-custody death conditions have not been in life-threatening range. In their series, in which significant acidosis was detailed, Hick et al. comment that the highest potassium was only 6.0 mEq/L and most were between 3.5 and 4.5. Therefore, at least from what limited data we have, hyperkalemia does not seem to be a major contributing factor to why these individuals die.

## *Respiratory Effects*

Just as the abruptness of the deaths suggests that cardiac dysfunction should be considered an etiology of death in individuals suffering sudden in-custody death, likewise respiratory dysfunction should also be considered. However, at least from the contribution of illicit drug use, there is little if any data to support a hypothesis that sympathomimetic drug effects may have an adverse impact that could contribute to respiratory dysfunction as a mechanism of death in restraint. Various pulmonary effects of particularly smoking cocaine have been reported *(61)*. However, autopsies have not revealed pulmonary abnormalities associated with chronic cocaine use. As addressed in other parts of this book the whole concept of these deaths being associated with respiratory compromise at all is not well supported.

## FORENSIC DRUG TESTING IN THE SETTING OF SUDDEN IN-CUSTODY DEATH

All individuals who die from sudden in-custody death syndrome should have toxicological testing performed because of the strong association with the use of certain illicit drugs. Ideally, all of the sympathomimetic drugs, including cocaine, methamphetamine, PCP, and LSD, that have classically been associated with this syndrome should be tested for their presence. Additionally, the major metabolites of cocaine and methamphetamine, benzoylecgonine, and amphetamine, respectively, should also be tested for their presence. If there is concern for the use of other illicit or licit sympathomimetic medications, particularly various amphetamines, they should be tested for as well. Examples include 3,4-methylenedioxymethamphetamine (ecstasy) and ephedrine. Although sudden in-custody deaths have not been widely reported with these other agents, based on their similarities to methamphetamine it is likely that they could be in the future. Interpretation of the results of toxicology screening in these cases should be left to those with experience in this field.

## TREATMENT

The key to treatment of individuals under the influence of illicit sympathomimetic agents who are in custody is prevention. Individuals experiencing toxin-induced excited delirium are dangerous not only to themselves, but others, and frequently require restraint. Even with the risk of sudden death in these cases, the risks of nonrestraint may be greater. Therefore, prevention of death during and after restraint is most important, although in some cases may in fact be unavoidable. Getting patients with excited delirium to health care providers should be accomplished as soon as possible.

Patients entering the emergency department with excited delirium should be recognized as at risk for sudden death and evaluated immediately. The agitation of the individual often will preclude the ability of even checking vital signs, let alone placing the individual on monitoring devices and establishing intravenous access. Additionally, the risk of needlestick injuries from attempting to establish intravenous access on an agitated patient is not an inconsequential risk to health care providers. Therefore, the rapid administration of chemical sedation by the intramuscular route when the intravenous route is too dangerous, or not established, is the preferred method for controlling these patients.

Controversy exists regarding the ideal agent or combination of agents to administer to agitated patients. Both benzodiazepines such as lorazepam and dopamine antagonists such as droperidol and haloperidol are effective chemical restraint medications that can be administered by the intramuscular route. The dopamine antagonists are appealing medications since they antagonize the central nervous system dopamine agonism that characterizes intoxication with cocaine and methamphetamine. Both droperidol and haloperidol have the primarily theoretical risk of lowering the seizure threshold, and the exceptionally rare risk of precipitating torsade de pointes, a life-threatening dysrhythmia *(62)*.

Combining a benzodiazepine with either agent probably negates the additional risk of convulsions and is a common practice for many practitioners. Since convulsions are occasionally reported in those suffering sudden in-custody death, and can potentially worsen the pathophysiological state, benzodiazepine administration to all seems reasonable. All medications should be titrated to effect and may require repeat dosing. With regard to precipitating torsade de pointes, the risk to the patient and health care providers of inadequate immediate sedation seem far greater than the infinitely small risk of producing this dysrhythmia. Because of the effectiveness and rapidity of chemical sedation, this method should be investigated for prehospital use as well. Paralysis with neuromuscular blockers in exceptional circumstances where rapid chemical restraint is failing may also be considered, realizing that immediate airway support will be required.

When safe, and at the earliest opportunity, the individual with excited delirium should be placed on cardiac, blood pressure, and pulse oximetry monitoring, and intravenous access established. These individuals should be assumed to be hyperthermic and empiric cooling measures with mists and fans seems reasonable. Chemical antipyretics such as acetaminophen and ibuprofen are ineffective in decreasing sympathomimetic, or exertional-induced hyperthermia, and are unnecessary. When safe to do so, core temperature should be measured. Dehydration and rhabdomyolysis should also be presumed and administration of normal saline begun. The empirical administration of sodium bicarbonate is more controversial. Certainly, if severe acidemia is documented and suspected of contributing to instability, sodium bicarbonate should be administered. Additionally, for electrocardiographic findings such as QRS complex width prolongation, suspected to be secondary to sodium channel blockade by cocaine, sodium bicarbonate administration is indicated *(63)*.

## CONCLUSION

A clear, yet not universal association exists between the use of certain illicit drugs and sudden in-custody deaths. The drugs associated include cocaine, methamphetamine, PCP, and LSD. The exact role that use of these illicit drugs contributes to these deaths is not yet defined. Undoubtedly, use of the drugs at times precipitates an excited delirium that initiates contact with law enforcement. It is likely that the excited delirium itself combined with the other pathophysiological states that the drugs help produce, such as catecholamine excess, hyperthermia, metabolic acidosis, and convulsions, create a situation in which an individual is susceptible to sudden death while in custody or restrained. The particularly adverse cardiac effects of cocaine may help explain why it is the drug most associated with these deaths. Future research is needed to further define the contribution of illicit drug use to sudden in-custody death syndrome, and how they can be prevented.

## REFERENCES

1. Stephens BG, Jentzen JM, Karch S, Wetli CV, Mash DC. National Association of Medical Examiners position paper on the certification of cocaine-related deaths. Am J Forensic Med Pathol 2004;25:11–13.
2. Karch SB, Stephens BG. Drug abusers who die during arrest or in custody. J R Soc Med 1999;92(3):110–113.
3. Wetli CV, Fishbain DA. Cocaine-induced psychosis and sudden death in recreational cocaine users. J Forensic Sci 1985;30(3):873–880.
4. Stratton SJ, Rogers C, Brickett K, Gruzinski G. Factors associated with sudden death of individuals requiring restraint for excited delirium. Am J Emerg Med 2001;19(3):187–191.
5. Stratton SJ, Rogers C, Green K. Sudden death in individuals in hobble restraints during paramedic transport. Ann Emerg Med 1995;25(5):710–712.

6. Ross DL. Factors associated with excited delirium deaths in police custody. Mod Pathol 1998;(11):1127–1133.
7. Mercy JA, Heath CW Jr, Rosenberg ML. Mortality associated with the use of upper-body control holds by police. Violence Vict 1990;5(3):215–222.
8. Reay DT, Fligner CL, Stilwell AD, Arnold J. Positional asphyxia during law enforcement transport. Am J Forensic Med Pathol 1992;13(2):90–97.
9. Ruttenber AJ, Lawler-Heavner J, Yin M, Wetli CV, Hearn WL, Mash DC. Fatal excited delirium following cocaine use: epidemiologic findings provide new evidence for mechanisms of cocaine toxicity. J Forensic Sci 42(1):25–31.
10. Kornblum RN, Reddy SK. Effects of the Taser in fatalities involving police confrontation. J Forensic Sci 1991;36(2):434–438.
11. O'Halloran RL, Lewman LV. Restraint asphyxiation in excited delirium. Am J Forensic Med Pathol 1993;14(4):289–295.
12. O'Halloran RL, Frank JG. Asphyxial death during prone restraint revisited: a report of 21 cases. Am J Forensic Med Pathol 2000;21(1):39–52.
13. Mirchandani HG, Rorke LB, Sekula-Perlman A, Hood IC. Cocaine-induced agitated delirium, forceful struggle, and minor head injury. A further definition of sudden death during restraint. Am J Forensic Med Pathol 1994;15(2):95–99.
14. Pollanen MS, Chiasson DA, Cairns JT, Young JG. Unexpected death related to restraint for excited delirium: a retrospective study of deaths in police custody and in the community. CMAJ 1998;158(12):1603–1607.
15. Hick JL, Smith SW, Lynch MT. Metabolic acidosis in restraint-associated cardiac arrest: a case series. Acad Emerg Med 1999;6(3):239–243.
16. Park KS, Korn CS, Henderson SO. Agitated delirium and sudden death: two case reports. Prehosp Emerg Care 2001;5(2):214–216.
17. Andrews P. Cocaethylene toxicity. J Addict Dis 1997;16(3):75–84.
18. Hearn WL, Rose S, Wagner J, Ciarleglio A, Mash DC. Cocaethylene is more potent than cocaine in mediating lethality. Pharmacol Biochem Behav 1991;39(2):531–533.
19. Pudiak CM, Bozarth MA. Cocaine fatalities increased by restraint stress. Life Sci 1994;55(19):PL379–382.
20. Blaho K, Logan B, Winbery S, Park L, Schwilke E. Blood cocaine and metabolite concentrations, clinical findings, and outcome of patients presenting to an ED. Am J Emerg Med 2000;18(5):593–598.
21. Wetli CV. Fatal cocaine intoxication. A review. Am J Forensic Med Pathol 1987;8(1):1–2.
22. Karch SB. Interpretation of blood cocaine and metabolite concentrations. Am J Emerg Med 2000;18(5):635–636.
23. Davis AM, Natelson BH. Brain–heart interactions. The neurocardiology of arrhythmia and sudden cardiac death. Tex Heart Inst J 1993;20(3):158–169.
24. Pavin D, Le Breton H, Daubert C. Human stress cardiomyopathy mimicking acute myocardial syndrome. Heart 1997;78(5):509–511.
25. Wittstein IS, Thiemann DR, Lima JA, et al. Neurohumoral features of myocardial stunning due to sudden emotional stress. N Engl J Med 2005;352(6):539–548.

26. Wilkenfeld C, Cohen M, Lansman SL, et al. Heart transplantation for end-stage cardiomyopathy caused by an occult pheochromocytoma. J Heart Lung Transplant 1992;11(2 Pt 1):363–366.

27. Neil-Dwyer G, Walter P, Cruickshank JM, Doshi B, O'Gorman P. Effect of propranolol and phentolamine on myocardial necrosis after subarachnoid haemorrhage. Br Med J 1978;2(6143):990–992.

28. Drislane FW, Samuels MA, Kozakewich H, Schoen FJ, Strunk RC. Myocardial contraction band lesions in patients with fatal asthma: possible neurocardiologic mechanisms. Am Rev Respir Dis 1987;135(2):498–501.

29. Cebelin MS, Hirsch CS. Human stress cardiomyopathy. Myocardial lesions in victims of homicidal assaults without internal injuries. Hum Pathol 1980;11(2): 123–132.

30. Tazelaar HD, Karch SB, Stephens BG, Billingham ME. Cocaine and the heart. Hum Pathol 1987;18(2):195–199.

31. Mets B, Jamdar S, Landry D. The role of catecholamines in cocaine toxicity: a model for cocaine "sudden death." Life Sci 1996;59(24):2021–2031.

32. Vitullo JC, Karam R, Mekhail N, Wicker P, Engelmann GL, Khairallah PA. Cocaine-induced small vessel spasm in isolated rat hearts. Am J Pathol 1989;135(1):85–91.

33. Lange RA, Cigarroa RG, Yancy CW Jr, et al. Cocaine-induced coronary-artery vasoconstriction. N Engl J Med 1989;321(23):1557–1562.

34. Flores ED, Lange RA, Cigarroa RG, Hillis LD. Effect of cocaine on coronary artery dimensions in atherosclerotic coronary artery disease: enhanced vasoconstriction at sites of significant stenoses. J Am Coll Cardiol 1990;16(1):74–79.

35. Benzaquen BS, Cohen V, Eisenberg MJ. Effects of cocaine on the coronary arteries. Am Heart J 2001;142(3):402–410.

36. Wijetunga M, Seto T, Lindsay J, Schatz I. Crystal methamphetamine-associated cardiomyopathy: tip of the iceberg? J Toxicol Clin Toxicol 2003;41(7):981–986.

37. Wiener RS, Lockhart JT, Schwartz RG. Dilated cardiomyopathy and cocaine abuse. Report of two cases. Am J Med 1986;81(4):699–701.

38. Przywara DA, Dambach GE. Direct actions of cocaine on cardiac cellular electrical activity. Circ Res 1989;65(1):185–192.

39. Xu YQ, Crumb WJ Jr, Clarkson CW. Cocaethylene, a metabolite of cocaine and ethanol, is a potent blocker of cardiac sodium channels. J Pharmacol Exp Ther 1994;271(1):319–325.

40. Kabas JS, Blanchard SM, Matsuyama Y, et al. Cocaine-mediated impairment of cardiac conduction in the dog: a potential mechanism for sudden death after cocaine. J Pharmacol Exp Ther 1990;252(1):185–191.

41. Bauman JL, Grawe JJ, Winecoff AP, Hariman RJ. Cocaine-related sudden cardiac death: a hypothesis correlating basic science and clinical observations. J Clin Pharmacol 1994;34(9):902–911.

42. Bozzuto TM. Severe metabolic acidosis secondary to exertional hyperlactemia. Am J Emerg Med 1990;8(4): 369–370

43. Sejersted OM, Medbo JI, Hermansen L. Metabolic acidosis and changes in water and electrolyte balance after maximal exercise. Ciba Found Symp 1982;87:153–167.

44. Conlee RK, Kelly KP, Ojuka EO, Hammer RL. Cocaine and exercise: alpha-1 receptor blockade does not alter muscle glycogenolysis or blood lactacidosis. J Appl Physiol 2000;88(1):77–81.
45. Bethke RA, Gratton M, Watson WA. Severe hyperlactemia and metabolic acidosis following cocaine use and exertion. Am J Emerg Med 8(4):369–370
46. Crumb WJ Jr, Clarkson CW. The pH dependence of cocaine interaction with cardiac sodium channels. J Pharmacol Exp Ther 1995;274(3):1228–1237.
47. Leon-Velarde F, Huicho L, Monge C. Effects of cocaine on oxygen consumption and mitochondrial respiration in normoxic and hypoxic mice. Life Sci 1992;50(3):213–218.
48. Armen R, Kanel G, Reynolds T. Phencyclidine-induced malignant hyperthermia causing submassive liver necrosis. Am J Med 1984;77(1):167–172.
49. Rosenberg J, Pentel P, Pond S, Benowitz N, Olson K. Hyperthermia associated with drug intoxication. Crit Care Med 1986;14(11):964–969.
50. Liskow B. Extreme hyperthermia fro LSD. JAMA 1971;218(7):1049.
51. Kojima T, Une I, Yashiki M, Noda J, Sakai K, Yamamoto K. A fatal methamphetamine poisoning associated with hyperpyrexia. Forensic Sci Int 1984;24(1):87–93.
52. Callaway CW, Clark RF. Hyperthermia in psychostimulant overdose. Ann Emerg Med 1994;24(1):68–76.
53. Rockhold RW, Carver ES, Ishizuka Y, Hoskins B, Ho IK. Dopamine receptors mediate cocaine-induced temperature responses in spontaneously hypertensive and Wistar-Kyoto rats. Pharmacol Biochem Behav 1991;40(1):157–162.
54. Lomax P, Daniel KA. Cocaine and body temperature in the rat: effects of ambient temperature. Pharmacology 1990;40(2):103–109.
55. Marzuk PM, Tardiff K, Leon AC, et al. Ambient temperature and mortality from unintentional cocaine overdose. JAMA 1998;279(22):1795–1800.
56. Vescovi PP, Coiro V, Volpi R, Giannini A, Passeri M. Hyperthermia in sauna is unable to increase the plasma levels of ACTH/cortisol, beta-endorphin and prolactin in cocaine addicts. J Endocrinol Invest 1992;15(9):671–675.
57. Hanson GR, Jensen M, Johnson M, White HS. Distinct features of seizures induced by cocaine and amphetamine analogs. Eur J Pharmacol 1999;377(2–3):167–173.
58. Rowbotham MC, Lowenstein DH. Neurologic consequences of cocaine use. Annu Rev Med 1990;41:417–422.
59. Richards JR. Rhabdomyolysis and drugs of abuse. J Emerg Med 2000;19(1): 51–56.
60. Ruttenber AJ, McAnally HB, Wetli CV. Cocaine-associated rhabdomyolysis and excited delirium: different stages of the same syndrome. Am J Forensic Med Patho 1999;20(2):120–127.
61. Perper JA, Van Thiel DH. Respiratory complications of cocaine abuse. Recent Dev Alcohol 1992;10:363–377.
62. Richards JR, Schneir AB. Droperidol in the emergency department: is it safe? J Emerg Med 2003;24(4):441–447.
63. Wilson LD, Shelat C. Electrophysiologic and hemodynamic effects of sodium bicarbonate in a canine model of severe cocaine intoxication. J Toxicol Clin Toxicol 2003;41(6):777–788.

# Chapter 7

# Excited Delirium

*Charles V. Wetli*

## INTRODUCTION

"Excited delirium accounts for 1% of our EDP (emotionally disturbed persons) cases and 99% of our headaches." This comment, made some years ago at a New York City conference of police chiefs captures the managerial and legal concerns of this entity. Police managers are concerned because their officers are suddenly confronted with psychotic, violent persons, which sets into motion an escalation of the use of force continuum, and death may occur despite the appropriate application of sublethal control techniques. The violent nature of the conflict, often witnessed by citizens and sometimes the news media, often leads to accusations of excessive use of force by the police, which in turn may engender community outrage. Subsequent civil litigation against the municipality, the police department, and the individual police officers is to be expected.

Despite growing recognition of the hallmarks of excited delirium syndrome, some question the actual existence of this clinical entity. Although the National Association of Medical Examiners has recognized this syndrome for more than a decade, the American Medical Association does not recognize this diagnosis as a medical or psychiatric condition *(1)*. The American Civil Liberties Union contends that the syndrome is being exploited and used as a medical justification for excessive force *(1)*. This chapter reviews the history and clinical features of excited delirium, discusses related clinical syndromes as well as potential pathophysiological mechanisms, and presents a number of

From: *Forensic Science and Medicine: Sudden Deaths in Custody*
Edited by: D. L. Ross and T. C. Chan © Humana Press Inc., Totowa, NJ

case examples to illustrate this clinical entity associated with sudden in-custody death syndrome.

## HISTORY AND CLINICAL FEATURES

What we have come to understand today as excited or agitated delirium has a long history, and was first described by Dr. Luther Bell in 1849 *(2)*. Over the years, this entity has been variously known as Bell's Mania, acute exhaustive mania, and psychotic furors, among other terms. In a treatise on sudden death in psychiatric patients *(3)*, criteria for the diagnosis included extremely violent behavior with sudden death occurring while being restrained, the absence of drugs, and a "negative" autopsy. Although elevated body temperatures were frequently noted, hyperthermia was not required for the diagnosis. In the 1980s, the syndrome was recognized in cocaine users *(4,5)*. The typical victim was a young man with the sudden onset of paranoia followed by bizarre and frequently violent behavior. Jumping through a closed window or down an entire flight of stairs, inappropriate disrobing, smashing glass and mirrors, and running naked while screaming and sweating profusely were typical events. The screaming and shouting is often described as unintelligible or bizarre with religious or racial epithets, pleas for protection ("don't let them kill me"), or calls for the police despite the presence of several uniformed officers.

Bystanders or police officers who attempt to restrain the victim encounter violent, unexpected strength in a person who is totally impervious to pain that may be inflicted with compliance techniques, electric stun guns, or pepper spray. Typically, the victim continues to thrash about and struggle after being restrained. A sudden cessation of activity, sometimes interpreted as "playing possum," usually heralds a precipitous loss of vital signs. Medical responders (who are frequently already at the scene) find a lifeless person without any cardiac activity (asystole or pulseless electric activity being seen on electrocardiogram monitors). Should death be pronounced in a local emergency department after a period of attempted resuscitation, an elevated core temperature (average about 105°F) may be recorded *(6)* as well as a profound metabolic acidosis *(6)*. If cardiac function is restored, patients often subsequently die of multiple organ system failure and rhabdomyolysis within a few days of the initial cardiopulmonary arrest (Table 1).

It should be noted that, initially, the victim may alternate between periods of apparent normalcy and delirium. Also, the attempt to take the person into protective custody may be the trigger for the violent behavior. If these individuals are not taken into protective custody, they are in great danger of injuring themselves or others. They have been known to run into heavy traffic, attempt

### Table 1
### Common Presenting Features of Excited Delirium Syndrome

- Acute psychotic behavior
- Violent agitation
- Altered mental status and delirium
- Bizarre behaviors (e.g., jumping through windows)
- Profuse sweating
- Incoherent speech (screaming and shouting)
- Extraordinary strength and endurance
- Lack of response to painful stimuli
- Extreme exertion and hyperactivity
- Hyperthermia

to leap from one building to another, drown after running into canals or lakes, and so on. The dilemma facing police officers is, therefore, the real potential for serious or fatal injury if these individuals are not restarined vs the possibility of sudden death if they are!

It has been estimated that approx 10% of cases of excited delirium result in fatality *(7)*. The exact mechanism of death is not clear, and consequently, this fosters the environment for civil litigation because there is much to argue and little in the way of incontrovertible evidence. Simply put, some contend that the sudden death is the result of the extreme release of catecholamines, with or without the added effects of stimulant drugs, causing the heart to stop. Evidence for this includes observations that these are, indeed, cardiac deaths *(7)*, often accompanied by severe lactic acidosis *(8)*. Claims have also been made that death was the result of pepper spray or the application of an electronic stun gun.

Most often, the plaintiff allegation is that death was the result of "positional" or "restraint" asphyxia. This theory suggests that the method of police restraint interferes with the mechanics of breathing and the victim, therefore, suffocates. Currently, the main support for this theory is one of association *(9,10)*: because death occurs during restraint that seems to impair respiration, the death must be from asphyxia. However, there are now numerous studies that indicate the methods of police restraint, with or without pepper spray or pressure on the back, have nothing to do with the death *(11–16)*. Death has also been alleged to be the result of an improperly placed law enforcement neck hold (lateral vascular neck restraint or carotid sleeper hold) or outright choking. As is discussed further, neck injury must be interpreted with extreme care in assessing its role, if any, in the death of an individual with excited delirium.

RELATED SYNDROMES

As noted earlier, excited delirium has been previously described as "acute exhaustive mania" and "agitated delirium," and likely encompasses a group of entities best characterized as "acute excited states" *(17)*. Today, the entity is most common among chronic users of stimulant drugs such as cocaine and methamphetamine, and sometimes with LSD or phencyclidine abusers.

Although the syndrome of excited delirium is most commonly associated with drug use, the first cases of the entity were described in patients with underlying psychiatric disorders with no evidence of drug use, and in fact, prior to the isolation of cocaine from the coca leaf *(18)*. The National Association of Medical Examiners' position paper notes that "a catecholamine-medicated excited delirium, similar to cocaine, is becoming increasingly recognized and has been detected in patients with mental disorders taking antidepressant medications, and in psychotic patients (usually with a diagnosis of schizophrenia or bipolar disorder) who have stopped taking their medications" *(19)*. Although infrequent, excited delirium has also been seen in persons who, in retrospect, were developing schizophrenia but who had not yet been actually diagnosed as such and who were not given any psychotropic medications. Very rarely, excited delirium appears in previously mentally normal individuals who do not abuse drugs and whose psychotic break was precipitated by significant emotional trauma.

Because of similarities in clinical presentation, some have suggested that excited delirium is related to, or actually part of the spectrum of other syndromes, such as neuroleptic malignant syndrome (NMS) *(18)*. NMS is a disorder characterized by hyperthermia, altered mental status, and usually muscle rigidity. This highly lethal disorder has been associated with use of dopamine-antagonist agents (i.e., medications that block the actions of the neurotransmitter dopamine in the brain) often used to treat psychiatric conditions (neuroleptics). It has also been seen in individuals who are withdrawn from dopaminergic agents (such as levadopa and bromocriptine).

In addition, because of similarities in clinical presentation, excited delirium has been associated with the syndrome of cocaine-induced rhabdomyolysis *(19)*. Prior studies indicate that excited delirium accounts for approx 10% of all cocaine-associated deaths *(18)*. However, the clinical presentation of cocaine-induced excited delirium can be quite different from that of cocaine overdose. Ruttenber et al. compared 58 cases of cocaine-induced excited delirium deaths with 125 cases of death from cocaine overdose *(20)*. Compared with overdose deaths, the excited delirium deaths occurred more frequently in younger men and African Americans. Not surprisingly, because of the acutely psychotic behavior associated with excited delirium, more fatalities took place while in police custody. In addition, more of these deaths occurred during the warmer summer months when compared with cocaine-overdose deaths. Moreover, although evidence of chronic cocaine use was similar between the two groups (presence of the cocaine metabolite, benzoylecognine [BE]), individuals who died from excited delirium often had lower cocaine levels on autopsy when compared with cocaine-overdose deaths, suggesting that death in these cases was not caused by an acute, high dose of cocaine *(21)*.

## PATHOPHYSIOLOGY

Based on their study, Ruttenber et al. argue that "the toxicologic and epidemiologic data … suggest that a pattern of cocaine use characterized by repreated binges is associated with the development of fatal excited delirium" *(21)*. Although the exact mechanism of excited delirium remains unknown, a consensus is emerging among researchers that the pathophysiology involves the neurotransmitter, dopamine, and its effects on the brain. There is evidence that chronic cocaine use produces changes involving dopamine receptors, including decreases in the D1 dopamine-receptor subtype throughout the striatal reward centers of the brain, but do not affect the D2 dopamine-receptor subtype. This change likely represents an adaptive response (receptor downregulation) to increased intrasynaptic dopamine from chronic cocaine use, and may explain the fact that users quickly become tolerant to the drug's euphoriant effects. In addition, cocaine users have increased numbers of cocaine-recognition sites on the striatal dopamine transporter, suggesting greater ability to clear the increased concentrations of intrasynaptic dopamine *(21)*.

Individuals who suffer with excited delirium have been found to have significant differences in these adaptive responses to chronic cocaine use. First, there is evidence that persons with drug-induced excited delirium do not have an increase in striatal dopamine transporter sites in the brain, suggesting a decreased ability to clear dopamine from neuronal synapses *(21)*. In addition, these individuals have a decrease in D2 receptors particularly in the temperature-regulatory centers of the hypothalamus *(18)*. This decrease may explain the thermoregulatory abnormalities associated with excited delirium, particularly the malignant hyperthermia seen in these patients. Overall, individuals at risk for excited delirium may have limited compensatory mechanisms to respond to high levels of dopamine often precipitated by "binges" of cocaine and other stimulants. This vulnerability may then lead to the findings associated with excited delirium, including acute psychosis, autonomic dysregulation, and hyperthermia.

## CASE EXAMPLES

The following case descriptions depict examples of some of individuals with findings suggestive of excited delirium who suffered sudden death. The commentary at the end of each case emphasizes certain important aspects or nuances that may well be applicable to other similar cases.

### Case 1: Cocaine-Induced Excited Delirium

A 31-year-old man called his cousin to retrieve him from an alcoholic domestic situation. The two drove about for some time, occasionally consuming alcoholic beverages. The cousin stopped to make a telephone call, and the subject went to purchase some beer. Upon her return, the cousin saw the subject rigidly seated in the pick-up trunk, with a fixed stare, and unresponsive to her. As she began to drive, the subject began to hallucinate about streetlights and people climbing trees, and he perceived others were after him. He attacked his cousin, who stopped the truck and fled. She was again attacked by the subject, and citizens observing the incident called the police. A chase ensued and the subject attempted to break into an apartment. He confronted the police with a metal pipe, and several police officers swarmed him. Pepper spray and restraints about the ankles had no appreciable effect. With the help of nearby citizens, he was finally subdued, handcuffed behind his back, and his ankles were restrained. While the police were catching their breath, he was turned from a prone to a supine position, and found to be without vital signs. Cardiopulmonary resuscitation (CPR) was immediately initiated and when medical rescue arrived 3 to 4 minutes later, the subject was found to be in fine ventricular fibrillation. Resuscitative efforts were to no avail.

The postmortem examination revealed he was 66 inches tall and 185 lb. He had some external scattered abrasions and contusions. Petechiae of the eyes and lips were absent. Internally, there were scattered petechiae of the pleurae and epicardium, a minimally enlarged but otherwise normal heart, and no internal injuries. Toxicological analysis revealed blood concentrations of 0.01% alcohol, 0.35 mg/L cocaine, 2.4 mg/L BE and no cocaethylene (CE). Brain concentrations were as follows: cocaine, 1.2 mg/kg; BE, 1.4 mg/kg; and CE, 0.04 mg/kg. Death was attributed to acute cocaine intoxication. The plaintiff pathologist and police tactics experts both alleged the death was the result of "positional asphyxia," specifically because the subject was restrained in a prone position. The jury rejected the argument and returned a verdict for the defense.

### Commentary

The terminal events of this case are fairly typical for excited delirium regardless of the cause. In this case, the heart rhythm detected by medical rescue personnel was fine ventricular fibrillation, which is a bit unusual because most cases have asystole or pulseless electrical activity. A core body temperature was not taken, and this is needed to ascertain whether or not there was hyperthermia (palpation of the skin for body temperature in these cases is meaningless). Blood concentrations of cocaine and its metabolite, BE, are quite typical, the cocaine being usually less than 1 mg/L and the BE more than 1 mg/L, often with a BE to cocaine ratio of 5:1. In this case, the BE to cocaine ratio is 7:1. Brain levels are also of importance because they provide a better indicator of peak cocaine levels as a result of slower metabolism and because the BE in the brain is from cocaine in the brain (BE does not get into the brain from the blood). CE, a combination of cocaine and alcohol that takes place in the liver, is noteworthy in that it is directly toxic to the heart.

## Case 2: Delayed Death From Cocaine-Induced Excited Delirium

The police and medical rescue units were summoned to a residence because a 19-year-old male resident was hallucinating and intermittently violent. Nonetheless, upon arrival, the subject appeared coherent and, although uncooperative, was not violent. He eventually allowed his pulse and blood pressure to be taken, and the medical units departed. Shortly afterward, without provocation, he suddenly attacked the police officers. After a struggle, the subject was "handcuffed and hogtied" (i.e., ankle restraints were connected to the handcuffs by a strap) and he was taken to the local jail and placed in a restraint chair. It was noted that his "pupils were huge," he was sweating profusely, and he had a rapid pulse of 128 beats per minute (bpm). Notations and photographs taken of him in the restraint chair reveal he was hypervigilant and would generally become violent whenever somebody touched him. He sometimes exhibited aberrant head movements and would hyperextend his head.

Approximately 1 hour passed in the restraint chair before a nurse could draw a blood sample from him. Shortly afterward, he had grand mal seizures, and emergency medical responders (the same ones who were at the residence earlier) were summoned. He was found to have a blood glucose of 20 mg/dL. The seizures stopped with the administration of intravenous dextrose. At that time, his heart rate was 180 bpm and his blood pressure was 108 mmHg by palpation. He was transported to the hospital where, upon minutes of his arrival, his blood pressure was unobtainable, his heart rate was 40 bpm, and his core temperature was 108°F. Although resuscitative efforts restored cardiac function, he remained unconscious, developed rhabdomyolysis (massive breakdown of skeletal muscle), kidney failure, and disseminated intravascular coagulation. He died 1 week later. The blood cocaine concentration in the blood sample taken shortly before he had the seizure was 2.2 mg/L and the BE concentration was 7.2 mg/L.

During hospitalization, the subject developed a variety of pressure sores and other marks on the body from medical treatment. Plaintiff's experts, who took photographs while the subject was in the hospital, alleged these markings were injuries inflicted by the police and/or correctional officers and these in fact indicated he was killed by their actions. Fortunately, the hospital emergency department had a policy of photographing all injuries upon admission, and the pathologist nicely documented the true nature of the pressure sores and other marks. The jury concurred that the cause of death was complications of acute cocaine intoxication and returned a defense verdict.

### Commentary

The subject had many, but not all, the features of excited delirium. This is not unexpected because, with any syndrome, there is usually a wide variation in presentation. In this case, the subject exhibited violence, continued struggling while restrained, and had hallucinations and hyperthermia. The cause and role of hypoglycemia in this case are not clear. Cocaine levels were surprisingly high, but with a BE to cocaine ratio of about 3.5:1. Quite typically, initially successful resuscitation is thwarted by the rapid development of severe rhabdomyolysis (skeletal muscle breakdown), which releases myoglobin into the blood *(22)*. This leads to kidney failure, multiple organ failure, and other medical complications, which generally lead to death in a few days.

### Case 3: Methamphetamine-Induced Excited Delirium With Neck Injury

This subject had been drinking alcohol, "acting weird," and eating (presumably hallucinogenic) mushrooms one evening. Shortly after midnight, he jumped from the residence trailer to the outside. A friend followed him, tried to subdue him, and actually choked him with his hands. The subject broke his friend's grip, charged into a cement wall, and continued to yell and scream while running after he fell. At one point, he began to charge at his friend (who had pursued him) but suddenly changed direction and charged at police officers who had responded to the scene of a "fight in progress." During the ensuing struggle, pepper spray was used twice to no avail. A spit-hood was placed on him, and he was eventually restrained (maximum restraint or hogtied). His violent behavior continued during transport to the jail and in the jail as well. He finally became calm enough for removal of the handcuffs, however, leg shackles remained attached. A short time later he was noted to be in the same position, and inspection revealed the absence of vital signs. Upon arrival of emergency medical service personnel, he was noted to be pulseless, the cardiac rhythm alternating between pulseless electrical activity and asystole. Upon arrival at a local hospital, CPR continued, but to no avail. He was noted to have a blood pH of 6.6, and no elevation of cardiac enzymes or serum troponin.

The postmortem examination revealed a fractured hyoid bone and extensive hemorrhage into the neck muscles (from the earlier choking episode), the absence of petechiae, multiple contusions and abrasions, and an enlarged dilated heart with small caliber (hypoplastic) coronary arteries. Toxicology analysis revealed markedly elevated levels of methamphetamine (0.89 mg/L) and amphetamine (0.12 mg/L), a trace of propoxyphene, and no alcohol. Psilocin was not detected. Plaintiff's experts alleged that death resulted from "restraint asphyxia," with some also adding contributions by the spit-hood and the pepper spray (although it is hard to see how the spit-hood could impair breathing because most of it is comprised of a net). The original pathologist and defense expert pathologist attributed the death to methamphetamine toxicity with a contributory factor of dilated cardiomyopathy. The case settled out of court.

## *Commentary*

This individual exhibited most of the features of drug-induced excited delirium: paranoia, hallucinations, violent and aggressive behavior with unexpected strength, no reaction to painful stimuli (oleoresin capsicum [OC] spray, and choke hold in this case), and continued thrashing and struggling after being restrained. A severe metabolic acidosis with normal troponin is also typical. The mechanism of death in such individuals is the continued effect of the stimulant drug and catecholamines on the heart, coupled with a severe lactic acidosis from the struggle and hyperactivity. His underlying heart disease (dilated cardiomyopathy) provides an additional risk factor for sudden death.

Pepper spray is a severe mucosal irritant that some have alleged may cause respiratory embarrassment by constricting the bronchi (i.e., bronchospasm). However, this has never been reported in individuals with relatively normal lungs, and if it were to occur, death would be preceded by obvious respiratory distress, much like a severe asthma attack. Such did not occur with him. Also, delayed swelling of internal tissues of the neck from the irritant effect of OC spray did not occur, as demonstrated by the autopsy.

This case emphasizes that even a "striking neck injury" (the fractured hyoid bone and extensive hemorrhage into the neck muscles) must be interpreted with care. In this instance, there was never any allegation that the neck injury contributed to the death because it was known the subject continued to yell and fight long after the injury occurred, and the autopsy did not disclose any petechiae or internal swelling of neck structures. The main lesson is that neck injury, by itself, does not indicate a cause of death. Like any other finding at autopsy, it must be interpreted in the light of terminal events and other autopsy findings.

## Case 4: Acute-Onset Mental Illness and Excited Delirium

A 48-year-old, deeply religious Christian man with no significant medical or psychiatric history, and no history of alcohol or drug use, began exhibiting highly uncharacteristic and bizarre behavior. After failing to return from church one Sunday evening, he arrived at home 5 AM the next day fully dressed with a sports coat, but was not wearing shoes. He became combative, banging on the wall and yelling for his children to wake up. His bizarre behavior continued with extensive pacing around the house. His wife and others were unable to calm him, and he suddenly departed, still barefoot. Later that morning, he was driving his automobile west on a causeway when, at a very slow speed, he drifted over a curb and struck the perimeter wall of a restaurant. He exited the car and repeatedly claimed, "I'm Haitian." He resisted the attempts of responding police officers to restrain him, and this escalated into a violent confrontation with several additional police officers. During the prolonged struggle, he broke two sets of flex-cuffs before being restrained and put into a police car. At that point, he continued to kick and thrash about, broke another set of flex-cuffs, and struck his head on a plexiglas divider several times before finally being strapped in with a seat belt with his feet secured to a foot rest. He was seated upright and was being taken to the hospital unit of the county jail when he suddenly lost consciousness. He was immediately taken to an emergency department where resuscitative efforts proved futile and he was pronounced dead. Laboratory testing there revealed a hemoglobin of 9.8 mg/dL, a hematocrit of 25%, and a blood pH of 7.25. His core temperature 2 hours later was 102.1°F.

The postmortem examination revealed a black man who was 68 inches tall and weighed 203 lb. He had superficial abrasions, no internal injuries, and no petechiae of the conjunctivae or upper airway. He had a 500 g heart (enlarged) and mild coronary artery disease. Microscopic examination was confirmatory of the gross observations, and there was no evidence of a myocarditis or viral encephalitis. However, sickled erythrocytes were conspicuous in many of the histological sections. Toxicological analysis was negative for illicit drugs as well as medications. A neurochemical analysis of the brain revealed a marked reduction in the number of dopamine transporter sites. This finding would cause an elevation of levels of dopamine in the brain, which in turn contributes to psychotic and agitated behavior, and is also related to abnormal thermoregulatory function of the brain leading to hyperthermia (18,23). Death was attributed to acute exhaustive mania, and the manner of death was listed as natural.

This case generated intense community agitation and unrest with racial overtones. Indeed, the media even alleged that excited delirium/acute exhaustive mania was an "invention" to prevent lawsuits against the police. Besides a thorough investigation and meetings with community leaders and family members, the dopamine transporter studies of the brain gave objective evidence for a serious neurochemical abnormality in a previously mentally healthy man. The wrongful death action was dropped after the completion of discovery depositions.

## Commentary

Many prefer to use the term *acute exhaustive mania* when there is no evidence of drug toxicity. However, whether the result of drugs or mental illness, abnormalities of dopamine transporter sites can be demonstrated on samples of frozen brain. The presence of sickled erythrocytes could have been listed as a contributory factor of death because sickling of abnormal red cells in sickle cell trait may occur during episodes of hypoxia or acidosis, and may be fatal by itself. Likewise, the enlarged heart could also have been listed as a contributory cause of death.

## Case 5: Sudden In-Custody Death Not Related to Excited Delirium

A 29-year-old African-American man was spotted by police who recognized him as a subject with an arrest warrant. He ran from the police as they approached. One officer caught up to him and placed a hand on his shoulder. The subject attempted to bite the police officer, who responded by spraying him with pepper spray. The chase continued into a wooded area where the subject was finally taken into custody. This encounter took approx 5 minutes. The subject was escorted out of the woods while cursing at the police and periodically going limp of his own volition. About 22 minutes later, he was transported to a local hospital. During the 2-minute transport time, he appeared to lose consciousness, whereupon the police vehicle accelerated into an emergency mode. At the hospital he was received without vital signs and resuscitative efforts were abandoned 29 minutes later. Arterial blood gas studies were not performed. However, a blood count revealed anemia, with a hemoglobin of 10.2 and a hematocrit of 32.9%.

The postmortem examination revealed a slightly enlarged heart (360 g) and no injuries or obvious disease process. Toxicological analysis revealed a blood concentration of 0.07% alcohol, 0.08 mg/L cocaine, and 0.18 mg/L BE. The concentration of cocaine and BE in the brain were 1.15 mg/kg and 0.57 mg/kg, respectively. Also, 0.10 mg of cocaine was found in the gastric contents. A hemoglobin electrophoresis revealed the subject had sickle cell anemia trait.

The cause of death was listed as acute alcohol and cocaine intoxication with a contributory cause of death of sickle cell trait with anemia. The manner of death was listed as "accident" because of the alcohol and cocaine.

A wrongful death suit was filed against the county and others, including the distributor and manufacturer of the pepper spray. For economic reasons, the latter two parties settled out of court. During the trial against the county, the plaintiff argued that the death was really the result of the pepper spray and "restraint asphyxia." The jury rejected the argument and returned a verdict for the defense.

## *Commentary*

Not all deaths that occur suddenly in police custody are caused by excited delirium. Almost invariably, such deaths involve a natural disease process, which may be obvious in some and quite subtle in others. The behavior of this particular subject was one of evasion and poor judgment. He did not have the violent and psychotic reaction and "superhuman strength" so typical of excited delirium. Other cases, however, have been typified by intense violence and even bizarre behavior, but they lack the hallucinations and psychotic expression of those with excited delirium.

The cocaine and alcohol concentrations in this subject are not likely, by themselves, to have caused his sudden death, particularly after more than 25 minutes had passed from the time of the initial encounter. A gastric level of cocaine is what would be expected from normal gastric secretions, as compared with the much higher amount to be expected if the subject swallowed some cocaine to avoid police detection. Because he was African American and had just experienced intense physical exertion, a hemoglobin electrophoresis was done, and this revealed sickle cell trait. Although normally a benign condition, it may result in sudden death in the presence of hypoxia or metabolic acidosis. Normally, sickle cell trait does not cause anemia, as was documented in the hospital laboratory report. Although it cannot be proven after death, the most likely cause of the anemia was another genetic trait, $\beta$-thalassemia, hence the wording of the contributory cause of death as sickle cell trait with anemia. The presumed mechanism of death in such individuals is that the red blood cells, because of the metabolic acidosis, suddenly deform into a sickle shape and can no longer carry oxygen.

## CONCLUSION

For more than 150 years, the entity we now refer to as excited delirium has been known to be fatal in a very high percentage of cases. The excited delirium syndrome manifests with bizarre, violent, and agitated behavior;

altered mentation and delirium; incoherent speech; hyperactivity; extreme endurance and unusual strength; and autonomic dysregulation including diaphoresis (sweating) and hyperthermia. Although excited delirium is most commonly precipitated by drug use, cases have occurred associated with psychiatric illness. Moreover, the syndrome is distinct and separate from fatalities owing to drug overdose. Deaths from excited delirium are associated with a number of factors. Although the exact mechanism continues to elude us, an emerging pathophysiology suggests abnormalities in the dopaminergic neurotransmitter system play an important role. Because of the behavior associated with excited delirium, death often occurs in police custody after a violent confrontation, and the mechanism of death is of intense practical interest. These are legitimate questions that deserve scrutiny to be sure, but the scrutiny must be based on sound, objective investigation with scientific support. Assumptions and "junk science" lead to specious theories and, sometimes, at least, to civil injustice. In the meantime, police managers must cope, police officers must act, and scientists must continue to investigate.

## REFERENCES

1. Paquette M. Excited delirium: does it exist? Perspectives in Psychiatric Care 2003;39:93–94.
2. Wetli CV. The history of excited delirium: characteristics, causes, and proposed mechanics for sudden death. In: Encyclopedia of Forensic and Legal Medicine, Elsevier, UK , 2005.
3. Wendkos MH. Acute Exhaustive Mania in Sudden Death and Psychiatric Illness, Spectrum Publications, New York/London, 1979, pp. 165–175.
4. Fishbain DA, Wetli CV. Cocaine intoxication, delirium, and death in a body packer. Ann Emerg Med 1981;10:531–532.
5. Wetli CV, Fishbain DA. Cocaine-induced psychosis and sudden death in recreational cocaine users, J. Forensic Sci 1985;30:873–880.
6. Raval M, Wetli CV. Sudden death from cocaine-induced excited delirium: aro-analysis of 45 cases., Am J Clin Path 1995;104(3):379
7. Stratton ST, Rogers C, Brickett K, GruzinskiG. Factors associated with sudden death of individuals requiring restraint for excited delirium. Am J Emerg Med 2001;19:187–191.
8. Hick JL, Smith SW, Lynch MT. Metabolic acidosis in restraint—associated cardiac arrest: a case series. Acad Emerg Med 1999;6:239–243.
9. O'Halloran RL, Frank JG. Asphyxial death during prone restraint revised—a report of 21 cases. Am J Forensic Med & Pathol 2000;21:39–52.
10. O'Halloran RL. Reenactment of circumstances in deaths related to restraint. Am J Forensic Med & Pathol 2004;25:190–193.
11. Chan TC, Vilke GM, Neuman T, Clausen JL. Restraint position and positional asphyxia. Am J. Emerg Med 1997;30:578–586.

12. Chan TC, Vilke GM, Neuman T. Reexamination of custody restraint position and positional asphyxia. Am J Forensic Med & Pathol 1998;19:201–205.
13. Schmidt P, Snowden T. The effects of positional restraint on heart rate & oxygen saturation. Am J Emerg Med 1999;17:777–782.
14. Parkes JM. Sudden death during restraint: a study to measure the effect of restraint positions on the rate of recovery from exercise. Med Sci Law 2000;40:39–43.
15. Chan TC, Vilke GM, Clausen J, et al. Related articles, links abstract: the effect of oleoresin capsicum "pepper" spray inhalation on respiratory function J Forensic Sci 2002;47:299–304.
16. Chan TC, Neuman T, Clausen J, Eisele J, Vilke GM. Weight force during prone restraint and respiratory function. Am J Forensic Med Pathol 2004;25:185–189.
17. Farnham FR, Kennedy HG. Acute excited states and sudden death. BMJ 1997;315:1107–1108.
18. Wetli CV, Mash DC, Karch SB. Cocaine-associated agitated delirium & the neuroleptic malignant syndrome. Am J Emerg Med 1996;14:425–428.
19. Stephens BG, Jentzen JM, Karch S, Wetli CV, Mash DC. National association of medical examiners positionpaper on the certification of cocaine-related deaths. Am J Forensic Med Pathol 2004;25:11–13.
20. Ruttenber AJ, McAnally HB, Wetli C. Cocaine-associated rhabdomyolysis and excited delirum: different stages of the same syndrome. Am J Forensic Med Pathol 1999;20:120–127.
21. Ruttenber AJ, Lawler-Heavener J, Yin M, Wetli C, Hearn L, Mash DC. Fatal excited delirium following cocaine use: epidemiologic findings provide new evidence for mechanisms of cocaine toxicity. J Forensic Sci 1997;42:25–31.
22. Roth MD, Alarcon FJ, Fernandez JA, et al. Acute rhabdomyolysis associated with cocaine iintoxication, N Engl J Med 1988;931:673–677.
23. Mash DC. Neuropsychiatric consequence of chronic cocaine abuse. In: Karch SB, ed. Drug-Abuse Handbook CRC Press, Boca Raton, FL, 1998, pp. 412–419.

# Chapter 8

# Riot Control Agents, Tasers, and Other Less Lethal Weapons

*Christian Sloane and Gary M. Vilke*

## INTRODUCTION

Less lethal weapons have become increasingly popular for law enforcement use when confronting dangerous, combative individuals in the field. On the use-of-force continuum, these technologies occupy an intermediate level between verbal and physical control methods and lethal force such as actual firearms. Less lethal weapons include riot control agents, electric stun devices such as tasers, and other blunt projectile weapons. Use of these less lethal technologies has been felt to increase both the safety of the intended target subject by supplanting the use of lethal force, as well as of the user by controlling and subduing dangerous, combative individuals. However, deaths have occurred in individuals following the use of such weapons, which were previously known as "less than lethal." A causal link between these various technologies and case fatalities remains controversial.

Riot control agents, such as tear gas, mace and more recently oleoresin capsicum (OC), have been used by law enforcement to subdue violent individuals or crowds. Other less lethal weapons becoming increasingly popular include the taser, other electric stun devices, and blunt projectile weapons used to control combative individuals while maintaining some distance between the subject and the officer. Many of these products, like mace, OC spray, and stun guns, have been modified by manufacturers to be marketed to the public and often are used by people with little or no training. Although generally safe,

From: *Forensic Science and Medicine: Sudden Deaths in Custody*
Edited by: D. L. Ross and T. C. Chan © Humana Press Inc., Totowa, NJ

there are precautions that should be used to maximize safety. In this chapter, the different types of riot control agents and less lethal weapons are discussed. This discussion includes their history, mechanisms of action, intended and other physiological effects, safety risks and complications, and potential association with sudden in-custody deaths. The associated research and case reports of injuries and deaths are reviewed in detail.

## RIOT CONTROL AGENTS

Riot control agents included a variety of substances that can be used to subdue individuals as well as large crowds. These agents include 1-chloroacetphenone (CN, trade name Mace), *o*-chlorobenzylidene malononitrile (CS), and OC ("pepper spray"). These agents are commonly dispersed as gases, smoke, or aerosols against individuals or large gatherings and, as such, may affect the user as well as the subject.

## CN (Mace)

### History and Properties

CN was first synthesized in 1871 by Graebe, and used in World War I. CN was the primary tear gas used by law enforcement and the military through the 1950s. This agent was also marketed for personal self-protection and was the product of choice until recently being replaced by OC sprays. CN is a colorless crystalline substance that can be disseminated in a smoke form from an explosive device, such as a grenade, or propelled as a liquid or powder. Harassing concentrations for CN are typically 10 mg/m$^3$ with the human LCt50 (concentration at which fatalities in 50% of those exposed would be expected to occur) estimated at 7000 mg·min/m$^3$ for pure aerosol and 14,000 mg·min/m$^3$ for a commercial grenade *(1)*.[1]

### Physiological Effects

CN acts as an irritant smoke when in contact with skin or mucous membrane tissues such as the eyes, nasal passages, oral cavity, and airway. Symptoms of exposure include coughing, sneezing, and increased airway secretions, as well as rhinorrhea and burning of the nasal passages and airways. Oral cavity and gastrointestinal exposure can result in the sensation of burning in the mouth, increased salivation, gagging, nausea, and vomiting. Ocular exposure to CN causes a burning sensation in the eye, injection of the conjunctiva, eye irritation, photophobia, and tearing. Similarly, skin contact can result in burning, irritation, and erythema.

## Case Reports

A prisoner was found dead under his bunk 46 hours after a "prolonged gassing" of inmates confined to individual cells with closed windows and doors and no ventilation. CN was used in the form of six thermal grenades, fourteen 100 g projectiles and more than 500 mL of 8% CS solution. The authors calculated the Ct to be 41,000 mg·min/ $m^3$. Details of other inmates' medical presentations were limited, but three were reported to require medical evaluation. The deceased inmate was found in rigor mortis and on autopsy was noted to have subpleural petechiae, hyperemia, mild edema, and patchy areas of consolidation in the lungs. His larynx, trachea, and bronchi were lined with an exudative pseudomembrane *(2)*. Another reported death occurred after exposure in a closed room with an estimated Ct of 142,500, 10 times the LCt50. The individual survived to hospital admission, but ultimately died 12 hours later. On autopsy, there were similar findings as with the previous case, including pseudomembrane formation along the bronchial tree and associated edema and inflammation of the walls as well as early patchy regions of pneumonia *(3)*.

One case series discusses the medical complications associated with prolonged exposure to CN in a prison incident. Surrounding circumstances include prolonged and recurrent exposures, and those that occurred in closed space with limited to no ventilation. Cutaneous complications included first- and second-degree burns over 25% of the total body surface area. Several patients required acute treatment with steroids and bronchodilators for laryngotracheo-bronchitis, but none reported any permanent medical issues. All ocular complaints were self-limited and there were no corneal injuries or permanent damage *(4)*.

A few cases of allergic reactions are reported, particularly in people who have a previous, even distant exposure in the past. A case of severe allergic reaction was reported in a military recruit who had been previously exposed to CN 17 years earlier, which had resulted in minimal itching at that time. He then went through the typical military CN training chamber in which he remained masked in the chamber for 5 minutes, then by protocol, removed the mask and exited the chamber. He developed generalized itching within minutes of exiting, which progressed over the next several hours to generalized erythema to all parts of his body except the face portion covered by the mask and his feet. He developed a fever to 103° and by 48 hours had diffuse vesication and edema, followed ultimately by desquamation of much of his skin. He improved over the next week *(5)*. Other cutaneous reactions have been reported as well *(6)*.

Ocular injuries have been reported with the use of CN, particularly when a tear gas cartridge is discharged at close range. In some cases, particles of agglomerated CN were driven into the eye tissue by the force of the dispersion device, most often a blast. In these cases, chemical reaction damage was noted over the course of months to years. These injures were considered different than blast injuries in which particles other than CN would have been implicated *(7)*.

## Research

There is limited research on the potential risks of CN and sudden in-custody death. As noted previously, most deaths reportedly associated with CN have evidence of significant airway and pulmonary injury on autopsy, suggesting that prolonged exposures to excessive concentrations of CN can cause significant respiratory damage and compromise.

In terms of other injuries, although permanent eye damage has been reported in conjunction with the use of CN at close range, it is challenging to separate out whether the damage is from the CN or the actual weapon itself. However, at harassing or standard field concentrations, there is no evidence that CN causes permanent eye injury. Human studies placing 0.5 mg of CN on the skin for 60 minutes caused irritation and erythema for all participants, as compared with CS, which had no effects when used in amounts of less than 20 mg. When the skin was moist, 0.5 mg of CN caused vesication, whereas this was not seen in exposure to 30 mg or less of CS *(8)*.

## CS

### History and Properties

CS is a riot control agent first synthesized in 1928 by Corson and Stoughton (the origin of its code name). CS replaced CN as the standard riot control irritant agent in the US Army in 1959. By the late 1950s, it had replaced CN in most law enforcement agencies in the United States as well because of its perceived improved effectiveness.

CS is a white, crystalline solid that is insoluble in water and only partially soluble in ethyl alcohol. Because of its low vapor pressure, CS is typically disseminated by dispersion of the powder or solution by explosion, spray or smoke. Harassing concentrations are typically 4 mg/m$^3$. Because of its insoluble nature, decontamination of buildings or other items after exposure can be challenging. CS also has a high flammability rating and has been noted to cause some structure fires *(9)*.

### Physiological Effects

The clinical effects that may be seen with the use of CS are similar to those of CN, resulting in irritation and inflammation of the skin, airways, and mucous membrane tissues on exposure. The effects typically start within minutes of exposure and will continue as long as the person is exposed to the material. The degree of symptoms tends to worsen based on concentration and duration of exposure, with mild exposure causing tearing, watery eyes, nasal discharge, and coughing. As the exposure increases, effects can worsen to gagging and vomiting, increased skin and mucus membrane burning, and subjective tightness in the chest. These effects improve after removal of the exposure and gradually resolve over 30 to 60 minutes, but some symptoms, such as skin erythema, may last up to several hours. Tolerance to CS has been demonstrated from prolonged or repeated exposures *(3,10)*.

CS has direct irritating properties to the skin. After minutes of exposure, a burning sensation may be noted, particularly over moistened or freshly shaven areas. This may lead to erythema, which will typically resolve 1 to 2 hours after exposure. However, if the exposure is with a high concentration of CS, under high temperature, or humid environmental conditions, severe erythema along with edema and vesication can follow. The time course of the development of vesicles can be delayed up to several hours, but typically occur within the first hour or so. During riots in Washington, DC in 1968, firefighters were often exposed to CS when they entered buildings in which the agent had been used. The movement of the firemen and use of water hoses re-aerosolized the material. These unintended exposures resulted in erythema and edema on the skin of a number of firefighters *(11)*. In workers with repeated exposure and sensitization to CS, acquired contact dermatitis has occurred, confirmed by skin testing. Symptoms ranged from simple erythema to large vesicles and bullae. No pulmonary symptoms were reported *(12)*.

## *Case Reports*

After being exposed for 2 to 3 hours to CS tear gas canisters fired into a house, a 4-month-old infant required hospital admission for frequent suctioning of upper airway secretions. The infant was treated with steroids and antibiotics as well as positive pressure ventilation for respiratory distress and wheezing within the first 48 hours, and slowly improved until he developed a pulmonary infiltrate on X-ray. He required ventilatory support and ultimately was discharged home fully recovered after 28 days *(13)*.

Of nine marines involved with strenuous exercise and exposure to CS in a field-training exercise, several developed transient pulmonary syndromes, presenting with coughs, shortness of breath, and hemoptysis and hypoxia. Some required close monitoring and treatment for hypoxia, but all nine demonstrated normal lung function on spirometry, pre- and postexercise within 1 week after the exposure *(14)*. Hu reported a case of exposure in an individual with asthma who developed semi-chronic symptoms of cough and shortness of breath for up to 2 years after the exposure. Her forced expiratory volume in 1 second (FEV1) at 4 weeks postexposure was 62% of predicted and her forced vital capacity

(FVC) was 78%. At 18 months following exposure, her FEV1 was 128% of pre-dicted, with a 16% drop with brisk exercise in cool air *(15)*. Given the descrip-tion, it is difficult to determine if her subjective symptoms of dyspnea were related to her underlying chronic asthma rather than the CS exposure.

## *Research*

Although these reports suggest that exposure to CS could be lethal by potentially causing pulmonary damage, injury, and pulmonary edema, there have been no case reports of human deaths associated with CS use to date in the medical literature. Moreover, these reports indicate that pulmonary injury would only potentially happen at concentrations several hundred times greater than typical irritating or incapacitating doses *(16)*.

Moreover, there is little evidence that CS results in any permanent lung damage even after several exposures to field concentrations *(17)*. Bestwick et al. found no change in tidal volume, peak flow, or vital capacity compared to pre-exposure values when measured immediately and at 24 hours after exposure to CS in 36 subjects *(10)*. In another study on human subjects, Punte et al. reported that individuals subjected to daily exposures to CS (1–13 mg/m$^3$) showed no changes from pre-exposure levels of airway resistances measured 2–4 minutes after CS exposure, as well as on days 4 and 10 after exposure *(3)*.

In terms of other types if injuries, human studies have been performed to assess the effects of CS on skin using different concentrations and assessing the effects of various ambient temperatures and humidity levels. Subjects developed first- and second-degree burns at different levels and the authors concluded that many variables affect the likelihood of blistering, making risk assessment diffi-cult to predict *(18,19)*. Spraying 0.1 or 0.25% CS carried in different solutions into the eyes of humans caused inability to open the eyes for 10 to 135 seconds. Postexposure evaluation utilizing slit lamp evaluation noted a transient conjunc-tivitis, but no corneal damage *(11,20)*.

## *Oleoresin Capsicum Spray*

### *History and Properties*

OC sprays, also known as pepper sprays, are derived from the natural oily extract of pepper plants in the genus *Capsicum*. In the 1980s and 1990s, the use of OC spray by law enforcement agencies increased, as the use of CS was on the decline. By the 1990s, the majority of US states legalized the use of OC spray by the public *(21)*.

OC is made up of a mixture of fat-soluble phenols called capsinoids. Capsaicin typically makes up to 80–90% of these capsinoids and acts both as a

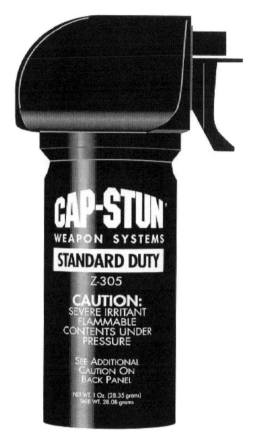

**Fig. 1.** OC spray. One example of OC spray device made by Cap-Stun, which delivers OC in an aerosol form.

direct irritant to nerve endings as well as stimulant for the release of peripheral neuropeptides. Other capsinoid analogues include nordihydrocapsaicin, nonivamide, dihydrocapsaicin, homocapsacin, and homodihydrocapsaicin. Capsaicin and dihydrocapsacin are the two capsaicinoids with the highest sensory values, which are typically expressed in Scoville heat units. The heat units were derived from an expert taste panel in conjunction with the Scoville Organoleptic Test, first employed in 1912 *(22)*.

The contents of different OC sprays vary depending on manufacturer and capsicum concentrations may range from 1 to 15%. Commercially available OC typically is about 1% in concentration. OC itself is not considered flammable. Delivery modes include liquid stream spray, aerosol spray, and powder delivered as a projectile (Fig. 1). The handheld stream or aerosol OC spray is delivered by a propellant at a distance of approx 5 to 15 feet. Other methods include delivery as an OC powder-filled projectile ball (Pepperball®) that is fired from a specialized launcher with a target range of 0–30 feet. When it hits the target, either the individual or a nearby object, the projectile ball breaks open and the powder is dispersed.

### Physiological Effects

Biochemically, capsacinoids stimulate chemonociceptors in primary afferent nerve endings, resulting in immediate pain and burning sensation over exposed areas of the skin, ocular, nasal, and oropharyngeal tissues. In addition, they cause the release of peripheral neuropeptides, including substance P. Substance P is a neurotransmitter that is involved in neurogenic inflammation and can cause vasodilatation, capillary leakage of plasma fluids, and pain sensation (23). OC spray can cause direct irritation to the eyes, skin, and mucous membranes. Onset of symptoms is almost instantaneous, causing burning and lacrimation of the eyes, as well as blepharospasm ranging from involuntary blinking to sustained closure of the eyelids. Cutaneous symptoms may include tingling, flushing, and intense burning sensation of the skin, particularly over recently shaved or abraded areas. Mucous membrane exposure, particularly of the nasal passages, will induce irritation, congestion, and rhinorrhea. Some subjects have complained of nausea as well. Exposure of the airway and respiratory tract to aerosolized OC may cause tingling, coughing, gagging, and shortness of breath. Some reports of a transient laryngeal paralysis with associated temporary inability to speak have also been reported (24).

### Case Reports

As OC spray is commonly used by many law enforcement agencies as a less lethal weapon, there are case reports and case series of deaths and injuries following OC use (24–27). Amnesty International claims that, since the early 1990s, more than 90 individuals have died following exposure to pepper spray in the United States (28).

Despite these reports, however, a causal connection between OC exposure and death remains controversial. In the early 1990s, Granfield reported 30 cases of in-custody death following OC exposure, in which drugs and underlying natural diseases were a significant factor in a majority of these cases (25). Pollanan reported 21 in-custody restraint deaths of which 4 of the subjects had been sprayed with OC (26). O'Halloran reported 21 cases of restraint in-custody death, of which 10 of the restraint episodes were preceded by use of OC spray (27).

In nearly all of these cases, OC was determined not to have been the cause of death. In only one case was OC implicated on autopsy. In that case, Steffee et al.

reported that a person who had a history of asthma and was sprayed with OC spray 10–15 times, suffered a sudden cardio-respiratory arrest. Autopsy revealed severe epithelial lung damage with the cause of death noted to be severe broncho-spasm probably precipitated by the use of pepper spray *(24)*.

Billmire reported a case in which a 4-week-old healthy male infant was sprayed in the face with a 5% OC spray when a key chain self-defense canister accidentally discharged. The child had sudden onset of gasping respirations, epistaxis, apnea, and cyanosis. The child required mechanical ventilation and ultimately extracorporeal membrane oxygenation. The child was discharged home after a 13-day hospitalization *(29)*. Four hours after exposure, an 11-year-old boy required intubation and ventilation for severe croup that resulted from intentional inhalation of OC spray. He was extubated 2 days later and recovered without sequelae *(30)*.

Other injuries that were not life-threatening have also been reported with OC exposure. As OC is commonly directed toward the face, symptoms often involve the eyes. Corneal abrasions have been reported in up to 8.6% of cases by Watson and 7% by Brown *(31,32)*. These findings have been noted as transient and do not require any additional treatment beyond decontamination with water irrigation. Vesaluma *(33)* also reported these temporary ocular injuries.

## *Research*

Because of its ability to block pain sensation and pruritis, presumably by depletion of substance P and other neurotransmitters, capsaicin has been studied in many different human clinical models, such as the treatment of various medical conditions (i.e., postherptic neuralgia, osteoarthritis, psoriasis, lichen simplex chronicus, diabetic neuropathy, and osteoarthritis). These capsaicin-related pharmacotherapies have typically been associated with topical application of the agent. Given its ability to induce coughing, capsaicin has also been utilized in many studies investigating the cough reflex and the pulmonary system, as well as to induce cough activity in order to assess the efficacy of various cough suppressants *(34)*.

Some animal and in vitro human tissue studies have suggested that capsaicin increases airway resistance and broncho-constriction *(35,36)*. However, clinical studies in humans with nebulized capsaicin are less definitive. Fuller reported that inhaled nebulized capsaicin resulted in a transient dose-dependent increase in airway resistance that was maximal at 20 seconds and lasted less than 60 seconds *(37)*. Blanc and Collier both reported no significant decrease in FEV1 in subjects who inhaled nebulized capsaicin at concentrations sufficient to induce cough *(38,39)*. However, direct broncho-constriction caused by capsaicin may be masked by cough and deep inhalation, because both have bronchodilatory effects.

In fact, subtussive doses of inhaled capsaicin have been shown to cause changes in airway resistance and pulmonary function *(40–42)*.

Unlike capsaicin, there is only limited research on the human effects of OC spray *(43)*. A number of observational reports have been published assessing safety of OC spray use. A 2-year joint study by the FBI and US Army reported that OC spray was not associated with any long-term health risks *(44)*.

Chan et al. conducted a randomized, cross-over controlled trial in 35 volunteer human subjects who were exposed to either OC spray or placebo propellant without OC, followed by a 10-minute period of being placed in either the sitting or prone maximal restraint position. During this time, pulmonary function testing was performed and arterial blood gases were monitored. OC exposure did not result in abnormal pulmonary dysfunction, hypoxemia, or hypoventilation when compared with placebo in either the sitting or restraint positions. However, there was an increase in mean heart rate and blood pressure in subjects exposed to OC that did not occur in the placebo group. The investigators concluded that OC spray did not result in any evidence of respiratory compromise with and without restraint that would make OC inherently lethal. The changes in cardiovascular parameters, however, indicated the need for additional study *(45)*.

Beyond research in the clinical laboratory setting, OC use has been widespread and a number of epidemiological studies have been reported on its use and safety. The California State Attorney General reported that no fatal consequences occurred in more than 23,000 exposures to OC spray. Watson et al. reviewed 908 exposures to OC spray in their region and found less than 10% of subjects exposed required any medical attention. Additionally, less than 1% complained of respiratory symptoms that required medical attention, and none of these were determined to have any significant injuries. There were no deaths reported in either of these studies *(32,46)*. Overall, OC spray has been used hundreds of thousands of times with no long-term health effects reported. Although there are case reports of death following the use of OC spray, other causes, such as drug intoxication, excited delirium, or underlying medical conditions, have been implicated as the primary cause of death, rather than the OC exposure, in the large majority of these cases. Moreover, clinical and epidemiological studies on OC have yet to report any compelling evidence that OC is inherently dangerous or lethal.

## Taser

### History and Mechanics

Taser is an acronym that stands for "Thomas A. Swift Electric Rifle" originally designed by John Cover, a NASA engineer and inventor. The name of the device is a reference to the Tom Swift science fiction series of the early part of the 20th century. The device delivers an electric shock or "stun" to incapacitate the subject. In the past decade, the taser has become the most popular incapacitating neuromuscular device on the market with an estimated 10% of all police officers in this country currently carrying the device *(47)*.

The taser was originally designed in the 1970s for airline personnel to use in the case of a hijacking. Law enforcement personnel subsequently adopted it in the 1980s and 1990s as an alternative to lethal firearms to subdue dangerous, combative individuals *(48)*. It is currently estimated that 30% of police agencies in the United States utilize the taser. As of October 2004, according to the Taser International® corporate website, tasers have been purchased by more than 6000 police departments in the United States and abroad. The manufacturer asserts that the device helps officers avoid the use of deadly force while lowering the risk of injury to officers. It has been used on more than 100,000 volunteers during training sessions in addition to more than 50,000 "real-life" police uses on subjects during field confrontations. The actual number of uses is unknown *(49)*.

Early tasers required officers to make close contact with subjects when discharging the device. These early tasers gained notoriety as the weapon used by the Los Angeles police to subdue Rodney King in 1992 *(50)*. Subsequent device modifications led to the development of current models that utilize barbs attached to wires. This new projectile design afforded the user greater safety and distance from the subject when utilizing this technology.

The progenitor of the modern-day Taser was developed by Taser International® with its first model, the Air Taser 3400, having the power of 7 W. However, early field-use trials demonstrated an effectiveness of only 86%. This led to the development of the Advanced Taser M26 with a power of 26 W, more than three times that of the Air Taser 3400 *(51)*. The most recent taser that has been developed and sold by Taser International® is the Taser X26. The X26 is a handheld device resembling a handgun that is intended to be used on subjects up to 21 feet away. It weighs approx 18 ounces, and is powered by either NiCad batteries or high-output alkaline Duracell ultra-batteries. The unit contains electronic circuitry, a laser light aiming guide, and two cartridges, one that is in position for deployment, and a second stored in the base of the handle in case the primary one fails. There is an on-board memory that saves the date and time of the last 585 most recent firings of the device. The energy output of the device is 26 W total, 1.76 J per pulse, 1.62 mA, 50,000 V. It uses an automatic timing mechanism to apply the electric charge for 5 seconds. When the trigger is depressed, a compressed nitrogen cartridge (1800 lb/in$^2$) fires two probes at an initial velocity of 180 feet per second.

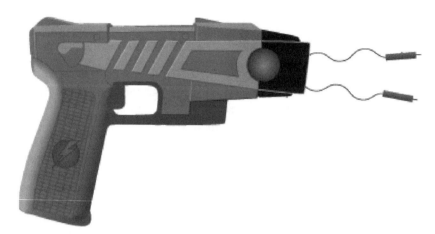

**Fig. 2.** Taser gun showing the device, its two probes, and the connecting wires.

The taser delivers its electrical discharge energy through a sequence of dampened sine-wave current pulses each lasting about 11 μs. This energy is neither pure AC nor pure DC, but probably akin to rapid fire, low-amplitude DC shocks. The electrical discharge is transmitted from the taser gun through thin copper wires to the end probes. The probes (also known as barbs or darts) consist of a thick metal base and thin metal shaft with a barb on the end (Fig. 2). They are designed to penetrate and stick in skin or clothing. The device will deliver its current and obtain the desired effect as long as the probes are within 2 inches of the victim's skin. The device may also be used in "drive stun" mode if the barbs and wires fail to function. The device is then used in the more traditional stun gun manner by holding the two electrodes against the skin of the target. Two types of the advanced taser exist. The police version can be deployed a distance of 21 feet, whereas the commercial version can be deployed a maximum of 15 feet. The manufacturer recommends 12–18 feet distance with the police model to obtain a 4-inch spacing of the darts that optimizes obtaining the desired effect.

### Physiological Effects

The current advanced taser works by incapacitating one's ability to maintain volitional control of the body by causing electrophysical, involuntary contraction of skeletal muscle tissue. It overrides the nervous system, resulting in loss of motor control by the subject. The advanced taser directly stimulates motor nerve and muscle tissue, causing incapacitation regardless of the subject's mental focus, training, size, or drug intoxication state.

Subjects report painful shock-like sensations with the feeling that all of the muscles in the body are contracting at once. During the tasering, subjects are unable to voluntarily perform any motor task, however, they remain conscious with full recall of the event. After the electrical discharged is halted, subjects are immediately able to perform at their cognitive and physical baseline.

The effects of tasers vary greatly, depending on the particular device used; location, placement, and distance between the probes on the subject's body and the condition of person at whom the device is fired *(52)* For example, probes that are located within a short distance on the body (less than 5 cm) will have less effect than probes further apart whereby the electrical discharge "stuns" a larger portion of the subject's body *(52)*. The effects of these devices have been reported to increase with the duration of application such that prolonged exposures may result in some sensation of fatigue and weakness even after the discharge is halted *(53)*.

A large number of police trainees have been tasered as part of their training in the use of the taser. One description reported that they remained awake and most felt "stunned" during the entire event and fell to the ground immediately. A few subjects reported a tingling sensation in an area approx 4 centimeters in diameter under the probe site that lasted 2 to 3 minutes after being tasered. Most reported that the experience was unpleasant and declined to be re-tasered *(54)*.

## *Case Reports and Reviews*

The use of tasers has been associated with cases of sudden in-custody deaths. There has been a great deal of publicity in the lay press recently regarding these devices, usually as a result of the death of a suspect on whom the device was used *(47)*. Amnesty International claims that more than 70 persons have died after being tased by law enforcement. However, a causal connection between tasers and these fatalities remains controversial.

Kornblum and Reddy examined 16 deaths that were associated with taser use during a 5-year period from 1983 to 1987 *(48)*. All involved young men with a history of abuse of controlled substances. All but 3 were under the influence of cocaine, PCP, or amphetamines. All were behaving in a bizarre or unusual fashion that necessitated calling the police. The ultimate cause of death was determined to be drug overdose in 11 of the cases. Other cause of death included three gunshot injuries and an undetermined death, In the 3 cases in which the individuals were not under the influence of drugs, 3 expired after being shot and another died after being placed in a choke hold.

There was one case in which the taser was felt to be contributory. In this case, the subject had a history of cardiac disease, for which it had been recommended that he get a pacemaker, but had not done so. On autopsy, he was noted to have a diseased heart, as well as lethal levels of PCP in his system. However, the cause of death was listed as cardiac arrhythmia owing to sick sinus syndrome, prolapse of the mitral valve, and electrical (taser) stimulation while under the influence of PCP *(48)*.

The authors concluded that the taser in and of itself did not cause death, but may have contributed to death in one of the cases. The authors suggest that the subjects in this study died after being in an agitated, manic, combative state known as "agitated delirium." Drug intoxication itself caused or predisposed the subjects to underlying vulnerability for sudden death, and the taser was not likely the causative factor.

These results were challenged by Allen, a pathologist in the Los Angeles coroner's department who was one of the actual pathologists on one of the cases studied. He criticized the authors' reporting of data, and conclusions drawn, suggesting that the taser was at least partly responsible for 9 of 16 of the deaths. "Obviously if a person is shot with a taser and then immediately killed with bullets, we are not in a position to draw a conclusion about whether the tasering was fatal. A similar consideration applies when forceful restraint or choke holds, which can also result in fatalities are used. My point is that, with more than one type of injury, we are not free to exclude the taser potentially contributing to death" *(55)*.

In a prospective case review conducted at the King/Drew Medical Center in Los Angeles from July 1980 to December 1985, researchers investigated 218 patients who presented to the emergency department after being shot with a taser. Data collected included age, gender, race, whether restraints were used, complications of the taser, and autopsy results if applicable. These patients were then compared with 22 similar patients who were shot by police with 0.38 caliber handguns during the same time period. Of all the cases in which the taser was utilized, 76% involved subjects displaying bizarre and uncontrollable behavior. Of these, 95% were men and 86% had a history of recent PCP use.

The mortality rate in the taser group in this study was 1.4% (3 of 218 patients). All three patients arrived to the emergency department in asystole or flatline on electrocardiographic monitoring. Taser probes were embedded in the thigh, buttocks, and back in these patients. All had high levels of PCP in their system. All three went in to cardiac arrest shortly after being shot by a taser, ranging anywhere from 5 to 25 minutes after taser deployment. The medical examiner's reports on all three cases listed PCP toxicity as the cause of death, with no signs of myocardial damage, airway obstruction, or other fatal pathological findings. When compared with the complications and injuries sustained from the 22 handgun shooting victims, the authors concluded that there is a marked and statistically lower rate of mortality and morbidity when the taser is used compared with the handgun *(56)*.

## Research

Research on the effects and safety of taser is limited. Most physiological investigations have been conducted in animal studies. In addition, the manufacturer claims no deaths have occurred as a result of thousands of uses on humans in the field setting as well as during training *(49)*. Definite research on the effects of the taser on human physiology is limited. In fact, the approval of the original devices was not based on actual human or animal studies, but rather "theoretical calculations of the physical effects of dampened sinusoidal pulses," for which the US Consumer Product Safety Commission concluded that the taser should not be lethal to a normal healthy person *(57)*. Understanding the effects of the taser on the various organ systems and physiology is critical to understanding the safety of these devices.

## Muscular Effects

The taser creates intense involuntary contractions of skeletal muscle, causing the subject to lose the ability to directly control the actions of their voluntary muscles. This is an electrical effect and it terminates as soon as the electrical discharge is halted. There is some residual muscle soreness reported by some who have been shot with a taser. There is no known permanent lasting effect on the muscular system aside from any injuries that may result from an associated fall.

Recent reports of an US Air Force study that was released to CBS news suggested that there was an elevation in the muscle enzymes creatine kinase and troponin T, both enzymes that are released during heavy exertion or muscle damage. Although the study is not available to the general public, a rise in these enzymes would not be unexpected, as the same increases would be seen in a person who had just performed heavy exercise, had a seizure with associated muscle contractions, or another cause for rapid, massive contraction or exertion of muscle *(47)*.

*Brain and Central Nervous System Effects.* There is no reported effect by the taser on the central nervous system. Subjects who are shot with a taser have complete recall, are awake and alert during the exposure, and resume normal control afterward. The discharge of the taser is painful and there may be some residual tingling at the site of attachment of the barbs. There have not been any published reports of seizures induced in either healthy or epileptic individuals by use of the taser. With regard to psychiatric disease, there have been no reports or studies on the possibility of the development or exacerbation of posttraumatic stress disorder or other psychiatric effects.

*Cardiac Effects.* The most commonly cited concern with respect to a relationship between tasers and sudden in-custody death syndrome centers on the possibility of the devices inducing cardiac dysrhythmias or cardiac standstill. The dysrhythmias or standstill would subsequently lead the heart to inadequately pump blood to the rest of the body inducing sudden death. The two main cardiac rhythm disturbances that are of greatest concern are ventricular fibrillation (VF), which is the unorganized or the lack of organized electrical activity and contraction of cardiac cells, and asystole, which is the absence of any electrical activity, commonly known as "flat-line."

For externally applied current like that of the taser, the chief concern is that of fibrillatory current, the current that produces VF. For externally applied current, the fibrillatory current in human beings is believed to be a function of the duration, frequency, and magnitude of the current, as well as the patient's body weight *(54,58,59)*. The threshold for VF in men for externally applied, 60 Hz current has been proposed to be 500 mA for shocks of less than 200 ms duration, and 50 mA for shocks of more than 2 seconds *(54)*. The longer a current flows, the greater the chance a shock will occur during the vulnerable part of the cardiac cycle, which is during early ventricular repolarization (first part of the T-wave on the electrocardiogram) and lasts for 10–20% of the cardiac cycle *(60)*. The Taser X26 carries a current of 2.1 mA for a duration of 0.0004 seconds *(49)*.

Additionally, resistance is also going to play a role in to how much current actually flows for a given voltage (Voltage = Current × Resistance). The lower the resistance, the larger the current that will flow and the more likely one will induce VF. The total resistance of the body is the sum of internal resistance plus twice the skin resistance as current enters and exits the body *(60)*. Current taser devices use very high-frequency electricity. A skin effect is known to exist when high-frequency electricity is used as these electrical currents tend to stay near the surface of a conductor. Hence, the output of the advanced taser is believed to stay near the skin and muscle surface of the body and not penetrate deeply to the internal organs, such as the heart *(61)*.

However, studies evaluating the effect of taser on cardiac physiology are limited. The majority of literature available for review related to cardiac effects is based on the older handheld models of stun guns or the early models of the Taser (M26). More recently, there have been studies that examine the current model of taser, the X26. However, most of these have been manufacturer-sponsored studies.

One animal study published in 1989 used an older model stun gun that produced high voltages (>100,000 V) and short-duration pulses (<20 μs). They used five different models of stun gun with varying energies. The average value of the current applied during each shock was calculated to be 3.8 mA, higher than the current value for the X26. When towels were placed between the skin and the electrodes (to simulate clothing), the maximum current spike was 190 mA with a pulse length of 20 μs. Using two anesthetized normal healthy pigs the investigators were able to induce VF when the leads of the stun gun were applied directly to the heart or to the chest of one of the animals in which a cardiac pacemaker was implanted. They surmise that the mechanism of action in that case was not to inhibit the pacemaker, but rather to allow the fibrillatory current direct access to the heart via the pacemaker leads. The shock also produced cardiac standstill when applied through the layers of simulated clothing for a prolonged period. However, these findings occurred with the two stun gun models delivering the highest energy. There were no cardiac effects seen with the lower energy units *(62)*. This study demonstrated that VF was indeed a possibility, but only at very high-energy outputs and when the electrical discharge occurred directly over or had direct access to the heart.

More recently, McDaniels and Stratbucker studied the Air Taser and Advanced Taser M26 in five anesthetized dogs with an average weight of 54 lb. Electrical discharge of the devices placed directly over the chest failed to induce VF. In 236 discharges, there were no recorded episodes of VF. The authors do note that when both probes were placed directly over the heart they were able to pace the heart similar to a pacemaker, but again did not induce VF *(63)*.

An unpublished study supplied by Taser International®, claims to demonstrate safety of the Taser X26, the model currently being marketed by the company. This study, performed on 13 adult domestic pigs initially used current applied to the thorax similar to that when the device is deployed on a human subject, and then gradually increased the energy output above that level until VF was achieved. The investigators did not induce VF in the pigs until levels of energy 20 times that of the standard level. When using energy levels below that threshold, 43 of 43 discharges did not induce VF *(64)*. This study suggests again that there is no cardiac effect in normal healthy animal hearts.

In another animal study, the cardiac safety of the devices was tested on nine pigs weighing 60 kg ± 28 kg. The animals were shocked using a device that was developed to deliver an electrical discharge identical in waveform and charge to that of the commercially available Taser X26 device. The voltage used for this study was less than the 50,000 V used in the device however. The animals were shocked for 5 seconds, simulating field use of the device. The electrodes were placed across the thorax of the animals using the barbs that matched the probes used by the standard device. The study used gradually increasing amounts of charge delivered to identify two levels. The first being the lowest amount of charge required to induce VF at least–once—the VF threshold. The second level defined was the highest discharge that could be applied five times *without* inducing VF—the maximum safe level. They then compared this value to the standard device discharge and the ratio of the two values, the VF threshold to the standard discharge was defined as the safety index.

The study found that the safety index ranged from 15 to 42 times the standard taser energy output as animal weight increased from 30 to 117 kg in a nearly linear fashion. In other words, the study found that the taser discharge required to induce VF was15 to 42 times the energy output of the standard taser discharge. This safety factor increased with the size and weight of the subject. The conclusions of the authors were that discharge levels output by field taser devices have an extremely low probability of inducing VF *(65)*. The authors contend that their results suggest it is unlikely that VF or cardiac dysrhythmias that are responsible for sudden deaths that have occurred after tasering.

Recently, Levine et al. conducted a study monitoring 24 subjects electrocardiographically immediately before and after taser shock during police training sessions. The investigators reported no changes in cardiac rhythm or electrocardiographic intervals following the taser discharge. Mean heart rate increased by just over 14 beats per minute following the taser shock, but no abnormal cardiac dysrhythmias were identified *(66)*.

The potential for inducing life-threatening cardiac dysrhythmias with current taser devices appears to be low based on these studies. However, there may be theoretical risks to patients with pacemakers or underlying cardiac disease, and the effect of recurrent or prolonged taser discharges remains unclear.

*Respiratory Effects.* There are no studies known to this date that focus directly on the taser's effect on the respiratory system. There are, however, studies that have examined the role of electric current on respiratory function. In rabbits, current applied to two limbs caused temporary or permanent respiratory arrest (possibly caused by cardiac arrest from prolonged respiratory arrest). A study of 60 Hz current in animals led researchers to propose a 40 mA asphyxia threshold *(54)*. The taser currently marketed falls below this threshold.

There is some theoretical concern that should respiratory function be inhibited, one could develop a respiratory acidosis as a result of hypoventilation *(52)*. This could potentially exacerbate any underlying metabolic acidosis from heavy exertion, drug use, excited delirium, or other reasons. The resulting severe acidosis or metabolic derangements could precipitate cardiac dysfunction. This is purely theoretical however, and is suggested as possible in part by the CBS news report of an air force study not yet available to the general public in which pigs were repeatedly subjected to multiple taser discharges. In the study, there was reportedly a decrease in pH similar to that seen with heavy exercise. The specifics as to the number of shocks, the devices used and the actual change in pH are not known. This is an area in which further research is needed.

*Other Physiological Effects.* There is a case report of miscarriage that occurred 7 days after being shot with a taser in the abdomen and leg *(67)*. In this instance, a 32-year-old woman who was approx 8–10 weeks pregnant was shot with a taser. One probe lodged above the uterus in the abdomen, and the other in the left thigh. Reports for the duration of shock varied from 3 to 10 seconds. The woman fell to the ground and was reportedly unable to move for 5 minutes afterward. One day later, she began having vaginal spotting that continued for 7 days. She later had increased bleeding and gynecological consultation diagnosed an incomplete miscarriage. Pathology analysis of the tissue from a uterine curettage revealed products of conception with extensive hemorrhage, necrosis, and inflammation. Although a temporal relationship is suggested between being shot by the taser and the miscarriage, no clear cause-and-effect relationship can be proven.

## Other Stun Devices

### History

Other electric stun devices utilized by law enforcement include the stun gun, electric shield and remote-activated custody control (RACC) belt. The US patent by Henderson and Williams in 1979 is the design from which most commercially produced stun guns are modeled *(53)*. Original stun gun designs centered on a handheld device that had two metal prongs sticking out from the end, which required constant contact with the subject being stunned in order to be effective. The use of this device meant that the person using the stun gun had to maintain close physical proximity to the subject on whom the stun gun was being deployed. Although painful when used, the device was easily overcome by those either highly motivated or under the influence of perception altering chemicals.

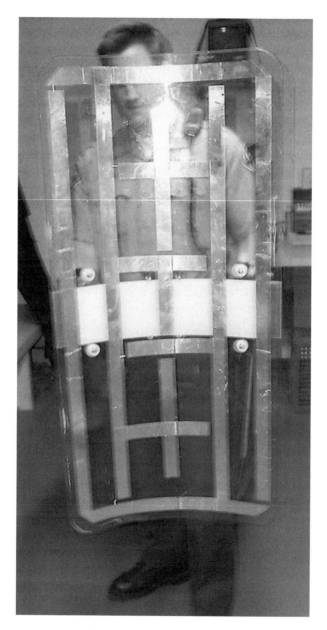

**Fig. 3.** Electric shield device.

The electric shield transmits 75,000 V across metal-conducting plates on a plexiglass shield that is pressed up against a subject (Fig. 3). This device works in the same fashion as handheld stun gun. The shield causes a noxious, painful stimulus when held in prolonged direct contact with the subject. The energies of this device are similar to those of handheld stun guns, namely 75,000 V, stun pulse rate of 17–22 pulses per second, and current of 3–6 mA.

The RACC belt (NOVA Technologies) is placed around the waist of prisoners in custody. It is remotely activated from as far away as 200 feet. Once activated, the device discharges for 8 seconds. The effects are like those of tasers. The energies of this device are similar to those of handheld stun guns, namely 50,000 V, stun pulse rate of 17–22 pulses per second, and current of 3–6 mA.

## Physiological Effects

The original stun guns worked by electrical shocks that stimulate sensory nerve fibers and cause significant pain. Focused or altered individuals could often overridethese weapons. The case of Rodney King is a prime example of why the weapons were not entirely effective. King was allegedly under the influence of PCP and even after two shocks of 50,000 V using the older handheld devices in drive stun mode, he was able to continue to resist officers. There have been no case reports in the medical literature describing death attributed to the use of the stun guns, electric shield, or the RACC belt.

### Blunt Projectiles

#### History and Mechanics

Blunt projectiles were first used during the Hong Kong riots of the 1950s and 1960s. Initial projectiles were made of wood. Similar devices were also used during the northern Ireland conflict and Israeli–Palestinian conflicts of the 1970s and 1980s. Early devices included hard rubber missile-shaped projectiles that were so inaccurate that hits to the head, face, and chest could not be avoided. Later versions evolved into PVC-type bullets, modern-day blunt rubber bullets, and bean bag-type rounds, which are currently in use by various law enforcement agencies in the United States. Although the specifics of each type of projectile are beyond the scope of this chapter, they all involve a blunt-type projectile that can impart energies on the order of 100–200 J depending on the type of round and the distance from firing at impact.

#### Physiological Effects

Blunt projectiles are used as an alternative to regular firearms when trying to disperse a crowd from a distance or when trying to subdue a combative, dangerous individual without the use of lethal force. The action of the blunt projectile is to induce pain, irritation, and often minimal injury to the subject without causing any life-threatening injuries that occur with the use of actual lethal force such as firearms. The physiological effects of blunt projectiles are directly related to anatomic location where the blunt projectile strikes the subject and induces blunt force trauma to the individual.

## Case Reports and Research

The association of blunt projectiles and sudden in-custody death syndrome mainly stem from risk of a direct blow to the chest inducing a cardiac dysrhythmia such as VF. This problem has a clinical name—*commotio cordis*—which is a rare, but reported syndrome in which apparently young healthy individuals suddenly suffer cardiac arrest after blunt chest trauma usually related to a sports activity (e.g., baseball, hockey, lacrosse, and softball). Commotio cordis is characterized by a sudden disturbance of cardiac rhythm in the absence of demonstrable signs of significant mechanical injury to the heart that is induced by a direct blow to the chest. This is separate from direct injury to the heart leading to myocardial contusion, valvular disruption, or pericardial effusion. Through animal studies, researchers found that impacts that were reliably timed to that part of the cardiac cycle that occurred between 30 and 15 ms preceding the peak of the electrocardiographic T wave were able to induce VF consistently. There is still debate, however, as to the precise pathophysiological mechanisms at work *(68)*.

The energies involved in the use of less lethal projectiles are on the order of the same energies that are involved in some of these different sporting events. Therefore, one could speculate that these devices would have the same risk of causing VF. As of the time of publication of this chapter, there have been no direct cases described of commotio cordis from flexible baton or bean bag rounds.

However, one specific case report of a death following the use of a blunt projectile was published in 1998. A 61-year-old woman was facing police in a threatening manner and was brandishing a butcher knife. After two unsuccessful deployments of a stun gun, the woman was subsequently shot in the chest using a plastic bullet (AR-1 baton round). She stumbled back and collapsed. She had labored breathing and subsequently suffered cardiac arrest. Autopsy showed she had sustained multiple rib fractures to the left chest, an underlying lung laceration, and heart lacerations that led to significant bleeding into the chest cavity. A tox screen was negative. The cause of death was certified as blunt force injuries of chest due to plastic bullet wound *(69)*.

Several studies have looked at the injury patterns from the use of plastic and rubber bullets. Their conclusions all tend to show that although generally regarded as less lethal weapons, significant injuries including death can occur when the weapons strike the chest, abdomen, or head. Millar et al. reviewed 90 patients who had sustained injuries to various parts of their bodies, concluding that the eyes, face, skull, bones, and brain are at greatest risk of injury from rubber bullets. The distance at which the rubber bullets resulted in serious injury ranged from 17 to 25 meters *(70)*.

Another study noted that of 80 subjects injured by rubber bullets, 4 died, 3 from ventricular dysrhythmias secondary to cardiac contusion and 1 from a hemopneumothorax (blood and air collapsing the lung in the chest cavity). Nineteen patients who required hospitalization had serious chest wounds. These investigators postulated a mechanism of injury involving shock waves producing shearing stresses and compression to soft tissue and bony structures resulting in contusions and fractures. Based on their finding, they state that any injury to the chest from one of these devices should be regarded as serious requiring close observation *(71)*.

## CONCLUSION

Riot control agents and less lethal weapons are criticized by some as inhumane and may be associated with sudden in-custody death syndrome. However, these agents hold an important role in the escalation of force continuum to maintain safety for law enforcement officers while offering the ability to incapacitate and mitigate at-risk individuals. These agents and weapons have saved countless lives by enabling law enforcement officers to avoid the need to use deadly force, and although, not truly "non-lethal," these less lethal agents have an overall excellent safety profile.

## REFERENCES

1. McNamara BP, Vocci FJ, Owens EJ. The Toxicology of CN. Medical Research Laboratories, Edgewood Arsenal, MD, 1968.
2. Chapman AJ, White C. Death resulting from lacrimatory agents. J Forensic Sci 1978;23:527–530.
3. Punte CL, Owens EJ, Gutentag PJ. Exposures to ortho-chlorobenzylidene malononitrile. Arch Environ Health 1963;6:72–80.
4. Thorburn KM. Injuries after use of the lacrimatory agent chloroacetophenone in a confined space. Arch Environ Health 1982;37:182–186.
5. Queen FB, Standler T. Allergic dermatitis following exposure to tear gas (chloroacetophenone). JAMA 1941;117:1879.
6. Madden JF. Cutaneous hypersensitivity to tear gas (choroacetophenone). AMA Arch Dermatol Syphilol 1951;63:133.
7. Levine RA, Stahl CJ. Eye injury caused by tear gas weapons. Am J Ophthalmol 1968;65:497–508.
8. Holland P, White RG. The cutaneous reactions produced by o-chlorobenzylidene malononitrile and 1-chloroacetophenone when applied directly to the skin of human subjects. Br J Dermatol 1972;86:150–154.

9. Danto BL. Medical problems and criteria regarding the use of tear gas by police. Am J Forensic Med Pathol 1987;8:317–322.
10. Bestwick FW, Holland P, Kemp KH. Acute effects of exposure to ortho-chlorobenzylidene malononitrile (CS) and the development of tolerance. Br J Ind Med 1972;29:298–306.
11. Rengstorff RH, Mershon MM. CS in Trioctyl Phosphate: Effects on Human Eyes. Medical Research Laboratories, Edgewood Arsenal, MD, 1969.
12. Shmunes E, Taylor JS. Industrial contact dermatitis: Effects of the riot control agent ortho-chlorobenzylidene malononitrile. Arch Dermatol 1973;107:150–155.
13. Park S, Giammona ST. Toxic effects of tear gas on an infant following prolonged exposure. Am J Dis Child 1972;123:245–246.
14. Thomas RJ, Smith PA, Rascona DA, et al. Acute pulmonary effects from o-chlorobenzylidenemalontrile "tear gas": a unique exposure outcome unmasked by strenuous exercise after a military training event. Mil Med 2002;167:136–139.
15. Hu H, Christiani D. Reactive airways dysfunction after exposure to teargas. Lancet 1992;339:1535.
16. Himsworth H. Report of the enquiry into the medical and toxicological aspect of CS (ortho-chlorobenzylidene malononitrile) II: enquiry into toxicological aspects of CS and its use for civil purposes. HM Stationery Office, London, 1971.
17. Blain PG. Tear gases and irritant incapacitants. 1-chloroacetophenone, 2-chlorobenzylidene malononitrile and dibenz[b,f]-1,4-oxazepine. Toxicol Rev. 2003;22(2):103–110.
18. Hellreich A, Goldman RH, Bottiglieri NG, Weimer JT. The Effects of Thermally Generated CS Aerosols on Human Skin. Medical Research Laboratories, Edgewood Arsenal, MD, 1967.
19. Hellreich A, Mershon MM, Weimer JT, Kysor KP, Bottiglieri NG. An Evaluation of the Irritant Potential of CS Aerosols on Human Skin Under Tropical Climactic Conditions. Medical Research Laboratories, Edgewood Arsenal, MD, 1969.
20. Rengstorff RH, Mershon MM. CS in Water: Effects on Human Eyes. Medical Research Laboratories, Edgewood Arsenal, MD.
21. Smith J, Greaves I. The use of chemical incapacitant sprays: a review. J Trauma. 2002;52:595–600.
22. Haas JS, Whipple RE, Grant PM, et al. Chemical and elemental comparison of two formulations of oleoresin capsicum. Sci Justice 1997;37:15–24.
23. Sanico AM, Atsuta S, Proud D, et al. Dose-dependant effects of capsaicin nasal challenge: in vivo evidence of human airway neurogenic inflammation. J Allergy Clin Immunol 1997;100:632–641.
24. Steffee CH, Lantz PE, Flannagan LM, Thompson RL, Jason DR. Oleoresin capsicum (pepper) spray and "in-custody deaths." Am J Forensic Med Pathol 1995;16:185–192.
25. Granfield J, Onnen J, Petty CS. Pepper spray and in custody deaths: international association of chiefs of police executive brief. Sci Tech 1994, pp. 1–8.
26. Pollanen MS, Chaisson DA, Cairns JT, et al. Unexpected death related to restraint for excited delirium: a retrospective study of deaths in police custody and in the community. Can Med Assoc J 1998;158:1603–1607.

27. O'Halloran RL, Frank JG. Asphyxial death during prone restraint revisited: a report of 21 cases. Am J Forensic Med Pathol 2000;2139–2152.
28. Amnesty International online at: web.amnesty.org (accessed March 28, 2005).
29. Billmire DF, Vinocur C, Ginda M, et al. Pepper-spray-induced respiratory failure treated with extracorporeal membrane oxygenation. Pediatrics 1996;98:961–963.
30. Winograd HL. Acute croup in an older child: an unusual toxin origin. Clin Pediatr 1977;16:884–887.
31. Brown L, Takeuchi D, Challoner K. Corneal abrasions associated with pepper spray exposure. Am J Emerg Med 2000;18:271–272.
32. Watson WA, Stremel KR, Westdorp EJ. Oleoresin capsicum (Cap-Stun) toxicity from aerosol exposure. Ann Pharmacother 1996;30:733–735.
33. Vesaluoma M, Muller L, Gallar J, et al. Effects of oleoresin capsicum pepper spray on human corneal morphology and sensitivity. Invest Ophthalmol Vis Sci 2000;41:2138–2147.
34. Foster G, Yeo WW, Ramsay LE. Effect of sulindac on the cough reflex of healthy subjects. Br J Clin Pharmacol 1991;31:207–208.
35. Lundberg JM, Martling CR, Saria A. Substance P and capsaicin-induced contraction of human bronchi. Acta Physiol Scand 1983;119:49.
36. Hansson L, Wollmer P, Dahlback M, Karlsson JA. Regional sensitivity of human airways to capsaicin-induced cough. Am Rev Respir Dis 1992;145:1191.
37. Fuller RW, Dixon CMS, Barnes PJ. Bronchoconstrictor response to inhaled capsaicin in humans. J Appl Physiol 1985;58:1080.
38. Blanc P, Liu D, Juarez C, Boushey HA. Cough in hot pepper workers. Chest 1991;99:27.
39. Collier JG, Fuller RW. Capsaicin inhalation in man and the effects of sodium cromoglycate. Br J Pharmac 1984;81:113.
40. Fuller RW. Pharmacology of inhaled capsaicin in humans. Resp Med 1991;85 (supp A):31.
41. Maxwell Dl, Fuller RW, Dixon CMS. Ventilatory effects of inhaled capsaicin in man. Eur J Pharmacol 1987;31:715.
42. Hathaway TJ, Higenbottam TW, Morrison JFJ, Clelland CA, Wallwork J. Effects of inhaled capsaicin in heart–lung transplant patients and asthmatic subjects. Am Rev Respir Dis 1993;148:1233.
43. Ross D, Siddle B. Use of force policies and training recommendations: based on the medical implications of oleoresin capsicum. PPCT Research Review 1996.
44. Onnen J. Oleoresin capsicum. International Association of Chiefs of Police Executive Brief, 1993:1.
45. Chan TC, Vilke GM, Clausen J, et al. The effect of oleoresin capsicum "pepper spray" inhalation on respiratory function. J Forensic Sci 2002;47:299–304.
46. Lundgren DE. Oleoresin capsicum (OC) usage reports: summary information. Report of the California State Attorney General, March 1996.
47. Hamilton A. From Zap to Zzzz. Time. March 28, 2005. Online at www.time.com/time/magazine (accessed March 28, 2005).
48. Kornblum R, Reddy S. Effects of the taser in fatalities involving police confrontation. J Forens Sci 1991;36:434–448.

49. Taser International website: www.taser.com (accessed March 28, 2005)
50. http://www.stun-gun-reviews.com/taser.html –(accessed March 28, 2005)
51. Griffith D. Electrical Storm. Policemag.com. 2002, 34–40.
52. Fish RM, Geddes LA. Effects of stun guns and tasers. Lancet 2001;358:687.
53. Robinson MN, Brooks CG, Renshaw GD. Electric shock devices and their effects on the human body. Med Sci Law 1990;30:285–300.
54. Koscove E. The taser weapon: a new emergency medicine problem. Ann Emerg Med 1985;14:1205–1298.
55. Allen T. Discussion of "Effects of the Taser in Fatalities Involving Police Confrontation." J Forensic Sci 1992;37:956–958.
56. Ordog G, Wasserberger J, Schlater T, et al. Electronic gun (taser) injuries. Ann Emerg Med 1987;16(1):73–78.
57. Obrien D. Electronic weaponry: a question of safety. Ann Emerg Med 1991; 20:583–587.
58. Ferris LP, King BG, Spence PW, et al. Effects of electrical shock on the heart. Transactions of the American Institute of Electrical Engineering 1936;55:498–515.
59. Kouwenhoven WB, Knickerbocker GG, Chestnut RW, et al. AC shocks of varying parameters affecting the heart. Transactions of the American Institute of Electrical Engineering (Communications and Electronics) 1959;78:163–169.
60. Forrest FC, Saunders PR, McSwinney M, Tooley MA. Cardiac injury and electro-cution. J of the Royal Society Med 1992;85:642.
61. Bleetman A, Steyn R, Lee C. Introduction of the taser into British policing. Implications for UK emergency departments: an overview of electronic weaponry. Emerg Med J 2004;21:136–140.
62. Roy O, Podgorski A. Tests on a shocking device—the stun gun. Med & Biol Eng & Comput 1989;27:445–448.
63. McDaniel W, Stratbucker R, Smith R. Surface application of taser stun guns does not cause ventricular fibrillation in canines. (unpublished data)
64. Stratbucker R, Roeder R, Nerheim M. Cardiac safety of high voltage Taser X26 waveform. (unpublished data)
65. McDaniel W, Stratbucker R, Nerheim M, Brewer J. Cardiac safety of neuromuscu-lar incapacitating devices. PACE 2005 1(suppl), s284–s287.
66. Levine S, Sloane C, Chan T, Vilke G, Dunford J. Cardiac monitoring of subjects exposed to electricity from the taser (Abstract). Acad Emerg Med 2005.
67. Mehl L. Electrical injury from tasering and miscarriage. Acta Obstet Gynecol Scand 1992;1;118–123.
68. Zangwill SD, Strasburger JF. Commotio Cordis. Pediatric Clinics of North America, 2004;51(5):1347–1354.
69. Chute DJ, Smialek JE. Injury patterns in a plastic (AR-1) baton fatality. Am J Forensic Med & Path 1998;19:226–229.
70. Millar R, Rutherford WH, Jonston S, Malhotra VJ. Injuries caused by rubber bullets: a report on 90 patients. Br J Surg 1975;62:480–486
71. Ritchie AJ, Gibbons JRP. Life threatening injuries to the chest caused by plastic bullets. BML 1990;301:1027.

# Chapter 9

# Case Analysis of Restraint Deaths in Law Enforcement and Corrections

*Darrell L. Ross*

The sudden death of an arrestee after a violent restraint altercation with the police or detention officers has emerged as a vexing problem, not only for the responding officers but also for the involved criminal justice agency, health care professionals, medical examiners, pathologists, the community, and the legal system. Such deaths have also occurred in psychiatric hospitals when staff members have been required to restrain a violent, mentally impaired patient. Although sudden in-custody death is rare in occurrence, the incident comprises a myriad of potential contributing factors that can make determining a cause of death problematic. Numerous questions of what contributed to the sudden death arise. These include the following:

1. Did the deceased contribute to his or her own death.
2. Did the individual die of a heart attack, heart abnormality, acute exhaustive mania, or asphyxiation?
3. Did the officers contribute to the death by use of the prolonged struggle and restraint procedures?
4. Had the subject been taking medication or abusing drugs, which over time rendered his or her heart more susceptible to cardiac arrest and sudden death?
5. Did the overwhelming emotional stress of the incident contribute to the individual's death?

Officers use the same physical control techniques and restraint methods or equipment thousands of times with varying populations without resulting in injury or death. Then, unexpectedly the same procedures are employed and a

From: *Forensic Science and Medicine: Sudden Deaths in Custody*
Edited by: D. L. Ross and T. C. Chan © Humana Press Inc., Totowa, NJ

person suddenly dies in custody. The death may result from reasons not related to the physical aspects of the confrontation or restraint. The death may have occurred from cardiac ischemia or failure, drug overdose, or other underlying disease of the subject. Frequently, however, autopsy findings do not reveal pathological evidence sufficient to fully explain the death. For example, not all neck trauma or conjunctivae/facial petechial hemorrhages indicate a death by asphyxiation *(1)*. Furthermore, placing weight on a violent, resisting person, restraining him or her with various devices, and placing the person in a prone restrained position does not in and of itself contribute to respiratory compromise *(2)*. Yet, a death certificate may still classify the death as a homicide because the restraining officers were the last ones to have contact with the decedent. Other contributing factors may also be attributed to law enforcement actions. For example, a death certificate may state that the primary cause of death was "cardiac dysrhythmia and recent drug use." However, it may also cite "restraint and positional asphyxia" as contributory. Still, other death certificates may identify the cause of death as accidental or undetermined, raising further questions directed at the actions of the restraining personnel, all leading to a lawsuit (*see* Chapter 11).

The problem is further compounded as pathologists and varying medical experts who examine the body, photos, tissue slides, and toxicology reports offer differing opinions as to the manner and cause of death. Although these "medical" opinions may differ, it is the responding officers, forced to make restraint decisions within seconds, without medical training, whose actions are frequently scrutinized and criticized.

Because these deaths often raise more questions than can be answered, examining the nature of these deaths through a case analysis becomes an important consideration. The purpose of this chapter is to provide an analysis of documented case reports that show the varying nature and circumstances of these deaths. Such an analysis can assist the medico-legal investigator charged with assessing these deaths and may enhance restraint personnel in developing practices and procedures in response to these encounters.

## PRIOR CASE ANALYSIS OF SUDDEN IN-CUSTODY DEATHS AFTER RESTRAINT

Since 1985, a limited number of medical and police studies have been designed to assess in-custody deaths, which comprise two common variables: "positional asphyxia" and "agitated/excited delirium." First, positional asphyxia deaths were believed to have occurred after a violent struggle and responding personnel maximally restrained the person in the hogtied position (wrists and feet mechanically restrained and connected together with a hobble, or other restraint device, with knees bent up) who suddenly becomes unresponsive and dies (*3–5*; *also see* Chapter 4, this volume). Second, deaths associated with excited delirium have been reported. Excited delirium deaths may result from cocaine psychosis (or other drug-induced delirium), acute mania, and acute psychosis (*6–11*; *see* Chapter 7, this volume). In the early stages, individuals become hyperthermic, extremely psychotic, and agitated with varying degrees of violence. Generally, they manifest great strength and a high threshold to pain. Owing to bizarre behavior, the police are contacted to subdue and restrain the individual as he or she becomes a danger to him or herself or others in the community

Wetli and Fishbain (*6*) reported the first known cases of excited delirium in-custody deathscustody. They reported seven recreational cocaine users who developed excited delirium; five died in police custody and three were placed prone in the hogtied position. All but one were men, exhibited blood cocaine levels ranging from 0.4 to 0.92 mg/L, and four had documented hyperthermia.

Wetli (*8*) reported such deaths associated with cocaine intoxication and acute psychotic reactions. Subjects came into police contact after exhibiting irrational behavior and continued to struggle with the police during and after being restrained. Wetli described the behaviors of these individuals as acutely paranoid, aggression toward glass, unusually strong, and hyperthermic. Frequently, these subjects died in the back seat of the police vehicle. Reay, Flinger, Stilwell, and Arnold (*4*) studied three deaths during police transport where all of the subjects were in a hogtied restrained position. These three male victims were taken into custody for violent and agitated behavior. Two had major psychiatric illness that explained the behavior and one was under the influence of alcohol, LSD and tetrahydrocannabinol. All three deaths were attributed to positional asphyxiation. The researchers noted the importance of performing scene and history investigation of the decedent, combined with a thorough autopsy and toxicological analysis. They also postulated a link between prone restraint and sudden death. McLaughlin and Siddle (*12*) were among the first to document five cases of custodial deaths in the police litera-ture. The major emphasis of the article dealt with an awareness of some of the risk factors associated with "sudden death syndrome" and the type of persons likely to be vulnerable to a death in custody.

In 1991, Kornblum and Reddy (*13*) studied 16 deaths of males in police confrontations where a taser was utilized. In every case, police encountered a call concerning a subject who was manifesting bizarre behavior. All but three of the fatalities had cocaine, methamphetamine, or phencyclidine in their blood at the time of death. Electrocution was not the cause of death in any of theses cases, and the authors theorize that the common factor in these deaths was the drug-induced state of bizarre behavior.

After five unexpected and sudden deaths in the San Diego area in 1992 *(14)*, the San Diego Police Department, in conjunction with the County Medical Examiner's Office, conducted the first national police survey of in-custody deaths. All of the individuals in the San Diego cases were men who demonstrated bizarre and violent behavior, exhibited signs characteristic of excited delirium, and fought with police officers. The subjects continued to struggle after being placed in prone restraint. Two were hogtied, two were strapped to a gurney, and one was handcuffed and placed in a prone position. In four of the cases, cocaine induced the psychosis, one case involved chronic schizophrenia, and one experienced a rapid pulse. Two of the men were sweating profusely and one was completely nude. In the national survey, data from the 142 respondent agencies failed to determine the frequency of occurrence of in-custody deaths, but it was reported that 43 agencies authorized using the hogtying method of mechanical restraint.

In 1993, O'Halloran and Lewman *(5)* studied 11 in-custody deaths related to excited delirium and restraint asphyxiation. All 11 were men, ranging from 14 to 44 years old. Each case revealed that the subject was in an excited delirious state and was restrained in a prone position. Three of the individuals were psychotic, whereas the others were acutely delirious from chemical substances (e.g., six from cocaine, one from methamphetamine, and one from LSD). Nine of the fatalities were in the hogtied position: two in the back seat of the police vehicle, five on the ground, and two on the floor. One was secured to a hospital gurney, and one was manually held prone. The authors discussed how subjects are more susceptible to sudden death during prone restraint when experiencing symptoms of excited delirium.

Mirchandani et al. *(15)* describe four deaths resulting from police restraint in Philadelphia. All subjects exhibited symptomatology of excited delirium, came into police contact because of bizarre behavior, struggled with police, and died. All of these fatalities had sustained a minor head injury after the onset of agitated delirium caused by cocaine use with or without other drugs. Toxicological findings revealed the individuals not only had cocaine or its metabolite, benzoylecognin in their systems but also had other drugs including morphine, methadone, diazepam, and codeine. They emphasize that all aspects of the death investigation be evaluated prior to making a definitive decision. In these cases, the head injury was insufficient to be the cause of death but rather drug intoxication played a more significant role in the sudden death.

In 1994, Granfield et al. *(16)* reported sudden in-custody deaths after exposure to pepper spray. These researchers noted 30 such incidents in 13 states between 1990 and 1993. All of the incidents involved male subjects and in none of these cases was pepper spray implicated as a cause of death. All of the decedents exhibited "bizarre" and combative behaviors at the time of police contact, the spray was ineffective in a majority of cases, subjects were restrained, and with one exception, all deaths occurred either immediately or soon after the confrontation. In 18 of deaths, positional asphyxia was cited as the cause of death, with drugs and/or disease as a contributing factor.

In 1998, Pollen et al. *(17)* reported 21 excited delirium-related deaths that occurred in Ontario Canada between 1988 and 1995. The incidents were indicative of the following: 12 subjects experienced excited delirium caused by a psychiatric disorder; 8 experienced cocaine-induced psychosis; 18 deaths occurred in police custody; 8 were restrained in the prone position and suffered chest compression; 4 were pepper sprayed; 4 had heart disease at the time of death; and none of the incidents involved a taser.

Ross examined 61 excited delirium sudden deaths in police custody between 1988 and 1997 *(18)*. He reported that all of the subjects fought violently with multiple responding officers, all were restrained, 23 were hogtied by police, and 9 were pepper sprayed. Impact weapons (including a flashlight) were used in 17 cases, and a neck restraint was used in 6 incidents. In 77% of the incidents, the decedent died on scene or during police transport and 66% died with 1 hour of police contact. The decedents were characterized as 97% men with a mean age of 32 years, mean body weight of 220 lb, mean heart weight was 405 g. Fifty-four percent were observed to exhibit seizure activity, 10% had brain abnormalities, and the mean body temperature was 104°F degrees. Cocaine was present in 69% of subjects (34% had cocaine and alcohol in their system) and 10% had other drug combinations noted on autopsy.

In 2000, O'Halloran and Frank *(19)* reported their assessment of 21 restraint deaths that occurred from 1992 to 1996 in the United States, primarily in California. A majority of the cases came to their attention through case litigation. The decedents were all male, age 17 to 45 years old, all were involuntarily restrained and held in the prone position, and four were hogtied. Eight of the decedents had a history of chronic mental illness and eight had a history of substance abuse. More than 80% *(18)* of the individuals appeared to be acutely delirious and exhibited signs of excited delirium, and 11 had stimulant drugs in their blood at autopsy. In 5 of the individuals, heart abnormalities were described. Death certificates listed asphyxia or a similar term in 13 cases and 8 listed drugs as a cause or contributory to death. The incidents involved the use of varying force equipment by the police: 4 were struck by an impact weapon, (2 of which were strikes to the head); 7 were pepper sprayed; and only 1 was tasered. None of these types of force applied were listed as contributory to the death of the individual. The manner of death was listed as accident in 14 cases, homicide in 4 cases, natural death in 2 cases, and undetermined in 1 case.

In 2001, Stratton et al. examined 18 deaths resulting from 216 arrests made of subjects exhibiting signs of excited delirium requiring restraint in Los Angeles from 1992 from 1998 *(20)*. They reported that all of the decedents violently fought with the police; 72% had heart abnormalities 72% had stimulant drugs in their systems, 56% had chronic disease, 56% were categorized as obese, and 28% were tasered.

There is increasing evidence that the stress of a restraint situation increases the probability of an in-custody death (*see* Chapter 5, this volume). Spitz *(21)* compared the restraint situation to "capture myopathy" reported in the veterinary literature, where death occurs in animals within minutes after capture. Studies conducted by Lown *(22)* and Engel *(23)* reveal the stress of perceived personal danger or threat to one's life produces a "fight-or-flight" mechanism conducive to lethal cardiac arrest.

Cebelin and Hirsch *(24)* reported death during assaults without a lethal injury. Hence, it is theorized that because many of the excited delirium individuals die after a period of struggle and restraint, the mechanism of death may involve a flood of catecholamines released by the stress response, superimposed on a myocardium already sensitized by cocaine *(25)*. The risk of sudden death is more pronounced after vigorous physical exercise. Mirchandani et al. also comment that physiological responses to stressful psychological factors may alone provoke sudden death and, when combined with drug-induced myocardial instability, there is even a greater likelihood of cardiac arrest *(15)*.

A significant report on this subject was conducted in 1996 by Ruttenber et al. *(25)*. They compared the victims of accidental cocaine deaths ($n = 125$) with excited delirium death decedents ($n = 58$) in Dade County, Florida from 1979 to 1990, and identified risk factors of excited delirium. Excited delirium fatalities more frequently expired in police custody, were male, black, younger (mean of 31.3 years), and had low body mass index (mean of 27.9). These victims also were more likely to have received treatment immediately prior to death, to have developed hyperthermia (mean of 104°F), to have survived for a longer period, and to have died in the summer months. Excited delirium victims showed clear evidence of behaviors characteristic of this disorder before encountering law enforcement personnel. Seizures were less frequently observed in the excited delirium group. The findings of this study reveal that excited delirium victims had concentrations of cocaine and benzoylecogine in autopsy blood that were similar for the control group. Study results support a hypothesis that chronic cocaine use disrupts dopaminergic function and, when coupled with recent cocaine use, may precipitate agitation, delirium, aberrant thermoregulation, rhabdomyolysis, and sudden death.

These studies indicate the potential lethality of cocaine and other drugs dating back for several decades. Research specifically examining deaths in police custody and excited delirium are more recent by comparison, owing largely to the recent deaths. A limited number of studies have reported on this phenomenon in arrest and restraint circumstances that pose an ongoing problem for the police and correction officers. These reports have begun to shed some light on this problem, indicating the need for further research.

## METHODOLOGY

The present research provides an analysis of deaths in police or correctional custody. Previous research has not specifically included incidents occurring in detention facilities.

Utilizing a content-analysis methodology, 145 case reports of a sudden in-custody death after a violent restraint incident were examined. The data sources for this analysis included incident reports from the police/detention officers, civil litigation documents, and autopsy reports. Sources of the data were collected from the police departments in which the death occurred by obtaining access to the legal division of the department and the medical examiner's office. The cases reviewed from 1995 to 2004 are representative of 58 agencies, 33 municipal police and 25 sheriff departments across the United States. Cases were obtained from the following regions across the country: western states (35%), central states (34%), northeastern states (18%), and southern states (13%).

Cases were considered for inclusion in the data set if they met the following definition adopted by Krosch et al. *(26)*: an unintentional death of an arrestee who exhibited violent and bizarre behavior where physical force measures or equipment were used by the police to subdue the person. The cases analyzed represent the following criteria:

1. The death resulted after an extreme violent struggle with responding officers.
2. The death resulted after responding officers force control and restraint measures were utilized.
3. The subject exhibited behaviors of excited delirium, induced by cocaine, other drugs, or mental disability.
4. The subject died on scene, during transport, at a confinement facility, or at the hospital within minutes or several days after the arrest incident.

The objective of this analysis was to examine five research questions:

1. What are the common decedent demographics?
2. What are the arrest circumstances commonly associated with these deaths?
3. What types of force measures are utilized by the police in these arrests and, what is the common location of death?

4. What are common causes of deaths attributed in these cases?
5. What are the common risk factors and descendant behaviors associated with   these deaths?

Common trends and patterns of theses incidents are presented. Case analysis examples of 13 incidents are also reported illustrating common patterns and findings. It is important, however, to note that this methodology represents a series of cases of sudden in-custody death, and does not account for the large numbers of individuals who undergo similar confrontations and restraint with police who do not die.

## FINDINGS

### Characteristics of Decedents

As illustrated in Table 1, the descendents were all men, 85% white, with an average age of 33 years, an average weight of 220 pounds, an average height of six feet, and a strong likelihood of a short survival time when in police custody. Ages ranged from 18 to 48 and the mean body temperature was 105°F.

### Table 1
### Decedent Characteristics (N = 145)

| Characteristic | N | % |
|---|---|---|
| **Race** | | |
| White | 85 | 59 |
| African American | 49 | 34 |
| Hispanic | 10 | 6 |
| **Seizures** | | |
| Unobserved | 97 | 67 |
| Observed | 45 | 31 |
| Unknown | 3 | 2 |
| **Survival time** | | |
| <1 hour | 97 | 67 |
| 1 to 5 hours | 5 | 24 |
| 6 to 12 hours | 10 | 7 |
| 2 to 3 days | 3 | 2 |
| **Mean age (years)** | 33 | |
| **Mean height** | 6 feet | |
| **Mean body weight** | 220 | |
| **Mean heart weight** | 425 g | |
| **Mean body temperature** | 105°F | |

The mean heart weight for males was 425 g and 20% had a brain abnormality (e.g., 10 with intrinsic lesions and 4 with gliotic scars).

Seizures or uncontrolled shaking were observed in 31% of the victims. The findings of survival time, age, and body temperature support previous research reported on this subject *(6–11,27,28)*. Slightly more than two-thirds of the deaths occurred within 1 hour after initial contact with the police. Death occurred 2 to 3 days after police arrest in three cases. Data of survival time was analyzed from the approximate time the police first encountered the individual to the recorded time of death, and does not reflect the actual time from the onset of delirious behaviors to pronouncement of death.

## Types of Drugs Associated With the Death

Table 2 reflects that the presence of various drugs in 69% of the fatalities (*n* = 100). Cocaine was the primary drug that contributed to the onset of excited delirium (59%). Blood cocaine levels ranged from 0.8 to 3.2 mg/L. Methamphetamine accounted for the second most common type of drug found followed by marijuana.

As shown in Table 2, decedents often consumed combination of drugs with cocaine or other drugs. The most common mixture discovered was cocaine and alcohol, considered to be a highly lethal cocktail. Benzoylecgonine, a metabolite of cocaine, was identified in 45% of the deaths. These two findings differ slightly from the Ruttenber et al. study *(25)* as blood concentrations of alcohol and benzoylecogine were moderately higher and reported more frequently in excited delirium victims in the author's study. A possible explanation for this factor variation may be attributed to the fact that the Ruttenber et al. analysis did not quantify benzoylecgonine for all decedents until 1990, which was the latter period of their study.

Other drug combinations are worth noting. Although blood levels of LSD were shown to be present in 19% of the cases, it was the sole drug consumed in seven cases and was combined with methylphenidate hydrochloride (Ritalin) in three cases, with marijuana in three cases, and combined with methamphetamine in one case. With the exception of lithium, valproic acid, and haloperidol, all other drugs were consumed with cocaine, and in a moderate number of cases they were combined with alcohol. Methamphetamine decedents also combined alcohol in 20 cases. In 5 cases methylphenidate hydrochloride was combined with alcohol and LSD. In 6 cases, traces of lithium were present and in 7 cases, valproic acid was also present in a manic-depressive individual. Valproic acid was also present in 11 other manic-depressive cases. Concentrations of haloperidol were present in 3 schizophrenic individuals. Presence of any concentration of drugs was absent in 45 cases.

Table 2
Type of Drug Consumed and Route
of Administration (N = 100)

| Drug type | N | % |
|---|---|---|
| Cocaine | 59 | 59 |
| Methamphetamine | 37 | 37 |
| Cocaine and alcohol | 56 | 56 |
| Marijuana | 49 | 49 |
| Benzoylecogine | 45 | 45 |
| Lithium | 30 | 30 |
| LSD | 19 | 19 |
| Valproic acid | 18 | 18 |
| Amphetamine | 17 | 17 |
| Methylphenidate hydrochloride | 12 | 12 |
| Haloperidol | 12 | 12 |
| Lidocaine | 10 | 10 |
| Phenylpropanolamine | 10 | 10 |
| Route of drug administration | | |
| Injection | 20 | 20 |
| Intranasal | 21 | 21 |
| Smoking | 10 | 10 |
| Ingestion | 9 | 9 |
| Unknown | 40 | 40 |

The route of administration for cocaine could not be determined in 40% of the cases. The primary route of cocaine administration was intranasal, which is consistent with the Ruttenber et al. study *(25)*. Autopsy records indicated old scars and needle marks in the arms of 45% of the victims.

Case examples 1 through 3 are illustrative of the encounters where varying forms of drugs were consumed by the decedent prior to the restraint confrontation.

## Case 1

Police encountered a 19-year-old white man who consumed marijuana, LSD, cocaine, alcohol, and methylphenidate hydrochloride (Ritalin) during a 24-hour period. He was 74 inches tall and weighed 175 pounds. Police responded to a call of a man running in the neighborhood close to a downtown college in the nude at 1:30 PM and acting psychotic. He violently fought with the two police officers. The officers applied two, 2-second bursts of pepper spray and struck him four times in the upper and lower legs, and shoulder area, with a flashlight, with no effect. He was finally physically controlled and handcuffed with hands behind his back. He died at the hospital. He sustained numerous abrasions to his body caused by running wildly in the neighborhood and fighting the police on the asphalt street.

The autopsy revealed a slight hemorrhage was noted on the right carotid sheath of the neck; there were no fractures to the hyoid bone, abnormalities of the heart, pathological lesions to the brain, abnormalities of the lungs or petechial hemorrhages. The rectal temperature was 104°F degrees. Toxicology showed 0.56 ng/mL of LSD, a blood alcohol content (BAC) of 0.27%, 2900 ng/mL of cocaine, and the presence of marijuana and Ritalin. The manner of death was categorized as homicide. The cause of death was classified as asphyxia due to neck injuries with multiple blunt force injuries to the extremities. Contributory causes were listed as acute drug intoxication.

## Case 2

A 37-year-old white male fought with five police officers and sent three of them to the hospital for treatment. He was partially clothed when the police confronted him in an alley at 4:30 PM. The officers struck him three times with an empty-hand strike to the side of the neck (Brachial Plexus Origin nerve), kneed him three times in the thigh of the right leg, and applied two bursts of pepper spray. The spray momentarily disabled him and he was physically controlled, handcuffed, and transported to jail. At jail he became self-injurious, began tearing up his cell, and experienced convulsions and seizures. Officers performed a forced cell extraction and removed him from the cell, and paramedics transported him to the hospital where he died 30 minutes after admission.

The autopsy revealed that he weighed 212 pounds and was 72 inches tall. There were superficial injuries on the face, neck, on the extremities, and on his back. The heart weighed 520 g and the left anterior descending coronary artery showed a 75 % anteriosclerotic narrowing. The brain weighed 1450 g and the cerebellum and brain stem were unremarkable. The right lung weighed 625 g and the left lung weighed 698 g. Rectal temperature was 106°F degrees. The manner of death was classified as undeterminable (drug abuse). The attending pathologist opined that he died of acute cocaine intoxication with no internal trauma contributing to his death, although there were superficial injuries to his external extremities. The toxicological report revealed cocaine levels of 13,763 ng/mL. Medical history showed he had a history of cocaine abuse for 10 years.

## Case 3

Police responded to a call concerning individuals fighting in a park at 3AM. One of the subjects became increasingly violent and fought with police.

After a short struggle and one burst of pepper spray, the subject was restrained in handcuffs. During police transport to jail he collapsed in the back seat. At the entrance to the police lock-up he was determined to be unresponsive and life saving efforts were unsuccessful.

The decedent was an African-American male, 43 years old, measured 68 inches tall, and weighed 170 pounds. The autopsy noted slight petechial hemorrhages in the right eye. There was bruising to the cheeks, dried blood in the nares, swelling of the nose, and palpable areas of swelling (knots) to the forehead. There was no evidence of acute external injury to the neck, chest, or abdomen. The laryngeal cartilages and hyoid bone were intact. There was no evidence of compression asphyxia or strangulation. There was no evidence of a skull fracture, brain swelling, or brain contusions. The brain weighed 1430 g, the heart weighed 390 g, the left lung weighed 500 g, and the right lung weighed 365 g. The toxicology report showed a BAC of 0.23, cocaine levels of 2900 ng/mL, benzoylecgonine of 2300 ng/mL, and cocaethlene of 600 ng/mL. The manner of death was classified as an accident and the cause of death was sudden cardiac death due to cocaine and ethanol induced excited delirium.

## Arrest Circumstances

Overall, 68% of incidents involved police officers responding to a violent subject and 32% occurred in a detention facility. Table 3 reveals that the most common police arrest circumstance was a disturbance call (41%). These types of police contacts involved the subject running in and out of traffic, wandering the streets, dancing or rolling in the street, destroying property in a house, hotel, or place of business, disorderly conduct in a public place (work, mall, or restaurant), and banging or kicking residence doors. Other police contacts were initiated by the subject driving a car erratically, assaulting neighbors or family members in a house or outside in the neighborhood, and attempting to break into a residence or business. Occasionally, the subject assaulted a friend with whom he or she had been abusing drugs.

The two barricaded house incidents involved mentally disordered subjects who had taken their family members hostage in their residence. One individual was schizophrenic and the other manic-depressive. Both individuals were experiencing auditory hallucinations. Police entered the residence after a reasonable period and the individuals violently fought with them. The subjects were subdued, restrained, suddenly experienced cardiac arrest, and died on scene.

## Use of Force Measures

Table 3 also shows the types of force measures police and detention officers used to control the subjects. All subjects were restrained with at least

**Table 3**
**Incident Circumstance and Force Measures Employed**
**by Police/Detention Officers (N = 145)**

| Incident circumstance | N | % |
|---|---|---|
| Disturbance call | 60 | 41 |
| Aggravated assault | 12 | 8 |
| Attempted breaking and entering | 10 | 7 |
| Operating vehicle erratically | 14 | 10 |
| Barricaded in house | 2 | 1 |
| Jail cell | 47 | 32 |
| Force measures used | | |
| Mechanical restraints | 145 | 100 |
| Empty-hand control techniques | 145 | 100 |
| Leg restrains | 96 | 66 |
| Hogtied | 28 | 19 |
| Impact weapon strikes/flashlight | 45 | 31 |
| Pepper spray | 105 | 72 |
| Neck restraint | 20 | 14 |
| Taser/stun gun | 30 | 21 |

handcuffs after a violent struggle. In two-thirds of the incidents, leg restraints were also used. Empty-hand control techniques were attempted or used in each incident, but because of the violent struggle and strength of the individual, the police had to resort to other force measures such as impact weapon/flashlight strikes, neck restraint, or taser. In the cases involving the taser ($N = 30$ cases), the cause of death was determined to be unrelated to the use of the taser. There were 105 cases where an aerosol (pepper spray) was used. Autopsy reports revealed that the spray was a contributing factor in two deaths. The totals in Table 3 for force measures employed do not add up to 100% as the police utilized a combination of force measures in one incident. On the average, the force confrontation required four officers to subdue and restrain the individual, ranging from three to six officers per incident. An additional restraining technique known as "hogtying" was used in 19% of the descendants because of the continued thrashing or kicking after the subject was handcuffed.

## Case 4

At 11:30 PM two police officers stopped a motorist who was driving his car erratically, crossing the center line several times. The officers approached the vehicle and observed that the driver placed his hand to his mouth as if to swallow something. One officer noticed a white/gray substance around the man's lips. The motorist would not exit the vehicle and he fought with the officers. A single short burst of pepper spray was applied and the subject exited the vehicle falling on one officer, pinning him to the ground. A violent struggle ensued and three more officers responded. The officers were able to restrain the subject in handcuffs and allowed him to calm down in a seated position outside the patrol car for 15 minutes. He was transported to the jail in a patrol car with the windows down. In the sally port he fought with detention officers and collapsed at the booking desk. There were never any signs of respiratory distress nor did the subject complain of medical problems while in police custody. Lifesaving efforts were unsuccessful and he was pronounced dead at the hospital. The officer who was pinned to the ground suffered injury to three disks in his back, required hospitalization, and received a medical retirement.

The suspect was a 36-year-old African-American, who measured 69 inches tall, weighed 402 pounds. Abrasions were found on both wrists. The brain weighed 1300 g, there was no brain edema, and the cerebellum and brain stem were unremarkable. The heart weighed 498 g and there was 75% narrowing of the coronary artery. There was no hemorrhaging of the tissues of the neck and the hyoid and cervical vertebrae were intact. The right lung weighed 580 g and the left lung weighed 390 g. Pulmonary edema was present and there was mucus in the airways, but there was no complete airway obstruction. The tongue showed fresh hemorrhaging. The liver weighed 2648 g, and the spleen weighed 227 g. The medical examiner opined that the manner of death was an accident. He further reported that the decedent died as a result of an acute bronchial asthma attack due to pepper spray-induced irritation of the airways. He developed acute brain anoxia resulting in cardiorespiratory arrest. Toxicology was positive for cocaine metabolites in the urine. There was no other trauma or natural disease contributing to his death.

## Case 5

Responding to a family disturbance call, three officers approached the porch of the house at 1 AM. The officers were on the porch when they heard a male voice state: "Get the f… out of here I have a hostage." Police were able to talk the man out of the house but he resisted once outside and two short bursts of pepper spray were used to subdue him. He was handcuffed and transported to the police station were he complained of breathing difficulties and then collapsed. Resuscitation efforts were unsuccessful and he died at 5:30 AM at the hospital.

The subject was a 25-year-old African-American male, who weighed 326 pounds and was 72 inches tall. The autopsy showed that the heart weighed

499 g, the brain weighed 1550 g, the right lung weighed 490 g, the left lung weighed 510 g, the liver weighed 2750 g, and the spleen weighed 300 g. There was no evidence of trauma to the neck and the hyoid bone and thyroid cartilage were intact. There was no airway obstruction but there was slight inflammation to the airway walls with mild thickening, a slight collection of mucus. There were slight abrasions on his right shoulder, right wrist, left medial elbow, and lateral left arm. There were no fractures to any of the extremities. His post-mortem BAC was 140 mg/dL (0.14%). Toxicology was negative except for caffeine. The attending pathologist concluded that the cause of death was asphyxia due to bronchospasm precipitated by pepper spray. The pathologist further concluded that the subject was predisposed to hyperactive airways and the temporal relationship between being sprayed with pepper spray, his respiratory compromise, and rapid demise all contributed to his death.

## Case 6

Two officers responded to a call of a partially clothed man ringing doorbells in the neighborhood, yelling, and kicking garbage cans down the street. The officers observed the subject and called for back-up. Two other officers responded and the officers attempted to calm him. The subject adopted a fighting stance and he was pepper sprayed with no effect. One officer deployed his taser and the subject pulled the barbs out of his sweatshirt. Another officer struck him twice with a baton. The officers were able to finally physically control him. He was restrained with handcuffs and one officer maintained control of him by keeping the his shoulders pinned to the ground. The officers noticed that the subject was unresponsive, began cardiopulmonary resuscitation (CPR), and had him transported to the hospital by emergency personnel. He died en route.

The decedent was a muscular white 31-year-old male. He was 75 inches tall and weighed 215 pounds. His right shoulder revealed purple abrasion marks from the use of the taser. Both wrists showed abrasions and there were contusions on his right thigh and hip area. There were no extremity fractures, and the neck did not show signs of trauma. The heart weighed 445 g, the right lung weighed 960 g, the left lung weighed 900 g, the brain weighed 1520 g, the spleen weighed 220 g, and the liver weighed 2170 g. There were mild autolytic changes present in the heart and congestion of the interstitial microvasculature. The brain did not show mass lesions, contusions, or inflammation. The toxicology report indicated methamphetamine was detected at a level of 0. 49 mg/L and amphetamine of 0.003 mg/L. The pathologist reported the cause of death as sudden death during restraint following blunt force trauma, taser application, methamphetamine intoxication with acute paranoia, and atherosclerotic cardiovascular disease.

## Case 7

Officers were sent to the location of a 911 hang up call at 11 PM. Once on scene, the responding officers learned that there had been a fight over a card game at a party. One of the male individuals began yelling profanities at the women in attendance and had chased them. A fight broke out between him and another male guest. The officers called for back-up and three more officers responded. They began to question the main fighter and he began yelling incoherently and kicked one officer in the ribs. A taser dart was deployed, but it was ineffective, and the officers physically restrained the subject in handcuffs. He was transported to the jail but would not exit the vehicle in the sally port. He kicked at the deputies. The taser was used again with no effect. Detention officers from the jail sprayed him with pepper spray, which had no effect on him. He was finally physically controlled and carried by four detention officers to a medical observation cell. As he was being examined by the jail nurse he went limp. Life-saving efforts were administered, an ambulance was summoned, and he was transported to the hospital, were he died.

The decedent was a 46-year-old African-American male, who measured 73 inches tall and weighed 180 pounds. There were several abrasions on his upper torso from the application of the taser, abrasions on the forehead, and eyelid. There was no skull fracture, intracranial hemorrhage, or brain injury. Both wrists had slight abrasions on them. There was no trauma to the neck or hyoid bone. The heart weighed 502 g with noticeable arteriosclerotic disease. There was 75 to 80% arteriosclerotic narrowing of the proximal, middle, and distal portions of the right coronary artery. The aorta showed moderate to focally severe arteriosclerosis. Pulmonary edema and congestion were present. The right lung weighed 870 g and the left lung weighed 681 g. Respiratory mucosa is congested and superficially ulcerated. Postmortem urine alcohol content was 0.31%. His lactic acids level was high. The attending pathologist concluded that the manner of death was natural. He died of metabolic acidosis with complications. Arteriosclerotic heart disease contributed to his death. The taser was not felt to be contributory to his death.

With some frequency, police officers have encountered a violent arrestee who is experiencing mental impairment who needs to be restrained. Commonly, the family has requested police assistance or a mental health hospital as the next two case examples illustrate.

## Case 8

At the family's request (the subject's sister), two officers responded to a residence to execute an involuntary commitment order issued by the court to transport the male subject to a private mental health facility for treatment. The man was diagnosed as bipolar disorder (manic-depressive). While in the house, the subject refused to cooperate and assaulted the officers by punching one in the face and kicking the other in the head. He threw an ashtray at one officer and hit one of the officers in the side of the thigh. Additional officers were requested, as was an ambulance. Three other officers responded and a struggle ensued. One officer struck the subject, by accident, in the head with a flashlight, and another officer punched him in the face. He was sprayed once with pepper spray, which assisted in allowing the officers to take him to the ground where he was controlled and restrained with handcuffs, with his hands behind his back. He was held down on the ground for about 2 minutes in order to calm down by two officers who held his legs and one officer who held his shoulders. Just as they were moving the subject up to a seated position, and as the ambulance arrived, the officers noticed that he was unresponsive. CPR was initiated and a slight pulse was discovered. During transport by paramedics to the hospital he became pulseless and he died as the ambulance pulled into the hospital's parking lot.

The decedent was a 41-year-old white man, with a long history of mental illness. He had not been taking his medications for about 3 weeks. He measured 77 inches tall and weighed 289 pounds. The autopsy showed that he had a laceration on his forehead, a cut lip, a broken nose, an abrasion on his cheeks, but no skull fracture, intracranial hemorrhage, or brain injury. The brain weighed 1589 g and there was no evidence of subdural hemorrhage. There were no fractures to the ribs or other bones. The neck was not injured but abrasions were found on the back. The heart weighed 510 g and the middle portion of the left anterior descending coronary artery had a small segment with 55% arteriosclerosis narrowing. The right lung weighed 810 g and the left lung weighed 725 g. Pulmonary edema and congestion were present, as well as large focal areas of autolysis. There was a small purple contusion on the upper chest area and acute congestion of the spleen. Toxicology was negative and the manner of death was ruled a homicide. The medical examiner opined that the decedent died of position/compression asphyxia with pulmonary edema. Acute psychotic reaction complicating chronic psychiatric disorder was contributory. He died during a prolonged struggle with several police officers.

## Case 9

Nursing and security personnel of a private mental health facility summoned the police to assist in controlling a combative patient. While family members were admitting the subject for treatment, he became violent, and assaulted a nurse and security officer. He was roaming through the facility damaging offices, computers, kicking walls and doors, and turned over a 55-gallon fish tank. Three deputies responded and encountered the subject in the hallway. He charged them and they sprayed three bursts of pepper spray with no effect. They summoned more back-up and two other officers responded. The subject left the facility to wash off the spray in the snow and then returned inside. Three deputies and two city officers confronted him in a hallway and they deployed two more bursts of pepper spray. This stopped him momentarily and he was brought to the ground. He struggled on the floor and the officers physically controlled and restrained him with handcuffs. He began to kick and they restrained his ankles with flex-cuffs. A facility nurse went to retrieve medicine for an injection but before she could return he became unresponsive. One of the deputies was cross-trained as a paramedic and began CPR. Paramedics responded and continued CPR and transported him to the hospital where he died within 15 minutes of arrival.

The decedent was a 42-year-white male who had a history of bipolar disorder. He had been awake for 38 hours prior to the incident and had become violent. He measured 79 inches tall and weighed 287 pounds. The autopsy showed that he had numerous abrasions on his hands, right side of the face, both shins, elbows, wrists, and ankles. There were no injuries to his head or skull. Examination of the neck showed a 2-cm contusion within the right side of the pharynx near the thyroid cornu. The neck did not show any natural disease. There were no fractures of the hyoid bone or thyroid cartilage. There was a 2- to 3-cm hemorrhage of right shoulder joint. The heart weighed 585 g and the aorta contained significant atherosclerosis. The right lung weighed 730 g, the left lung weighed 650 g, the brain weighed 1807 g, and the liver weighed 2965 g. One lung showed diffuse vascular congestion and there was pulmonary edema within some alveoli. A limited amount of conjunctival petechiae were noted in the eyes. Toxicological examination was negative. The manner of death was classified as an accident by the medical examiner. He also reported that the cause of death was positional asphyxia and acute exhaustive mania. Also contributing to the death was the man's markedly enlarged heart, which predisposed him to sudden death under stressful conditions. The pepper spray did not contribute to his death.

## Sudden Deaths in Detention

Table 3 also reveals that sudden deaths occur in detention facilities (32%). Detention officers can experience the same set of resistive behaviors that the police experience on the streets but because of the secure environment are limited as to the force equipment that can be used. Of the 47 incidents occurring in detention facilities, 87% of the detainees were psychologically impaired. A cell was the most common location for the confrontation, followed by the booking areas.

For example, after 3 hours of confinement, a prisoner experienced hallucinations and began destroying items in his cell and injuring himself by ramming his head into the cell bars. Officers entered the cell to restrain the prisoner. He violently resisted them for several minutes, and the officers finally used a neck restraint to subdue him, and placed him in a "four-point" prone position. Approximately 8 minutes later he was checked and found to be unresponsive and efforts of CPR were unsuccessful. He was pronounced dead at the hospital. Other detention cases were similar to the former, but lacked the mental disorder component. These involved cell rushes of the prisoners who were destroying items in their cells.

## Case 10

A schizophrenic detainee with hypertension and alcohol liver disease was being held at a jail for a probation violation. At 7:30 AM he refused his morning medications and began tearing up his bed, kicking the door, and flooding the toilet in the cell. A nurse responded with two detention officers to try and calm the prisoner and he threw urine at them. The jail doctor, who was his personal physician, tried to reason with him, but to no avail. The doctor instructed the jail commander to extract the detainee from his cell so that he could administer an injection. His cell door was opened and he charged the four officers. One officer sprayed one burst of pepper spray with no effect. The detainee knocked the officers into the hallway and fought with them. The officers were able to control him with handcuffs and leg irons. As the doctor began to administer an injection, he observed the detainee to be unresponsive. Life-saving efforts were unsuccessful and he died on scene.

The decedent was a 48-year-old white male who measured 75 inches tall and weighed 285 pounds. He had a history of mental illness and depression and was prescribed haloperidol and trifluoperazine. The autopsy revealed contusions on his face, left elbow, right-hand knuckles, both wrists, right foot, right knee, and both ankles. The heart weighed 510 g and the left anterior descending coronary artery showed focal calcific atherosclerosis with up to 50% reduction of the lumen. Examination of the heart also showed foci of fragmentation of the myocardial fibers, loss of striation, vascular congestion, and extravasation of erythrocytes. The right lung weighed 750 g and left lung weighed 720 g. Marked edema and congestion, with emphysema were noted in the lungs. Exam of the liver revealed alcoholic steatosis and hepatitis. There were no fractures to the skull or brain, and the brain weighed 1625 g. The toxicological examination was positive for acetaminophen, nortriptyline, metoprolol, and caffeine. The manner of death was determined to be natural. The pathologist ruled that he died of congestive heart failure during an anxiety attack owing to alcohol withdrawal syndrome. Hypertension and alcohol liver disease was contributory to his death. The restraint measures used by the detention officers were not felt to be contributory.

## Case 11

Two days after being confined in jail for malicious destruction of property and domestic violence, a detainee began fighting four detention officers after a recreational period. He kicked one officer in the groin and struck another in the face, breaking his nose. One officer sprayed one burst of pepper spray in the face of the detainee and two other officers took him to the floor. He struggled with the officers and was able to throw one off of him. One officer partially used a neck restraint only to control him. He was subdued, placed in handcuffs, and placed in an observation cell in four-point restraints, under medical supervision. Checks were made every 10 minutes for 50 minutes, when he was observed to be unresponsive. Life-saving efforts were unsuccessful and he died in the cell.

The decedent was a white man, very muscular, and a martial artist who was 35 years old, measured 75 inches tall, and weighed 215 pounds. The decedent had a history of mental illness for 16 years, and abused cocaine and alcohol. The autopsy revealed intravenous needle marks on both arms within the arm bends. There were abrasions on his right knuckles, on both wrists, and multiple linear abrasions on the back. There was no evidence of facial injuries but there was a slight cut on his lip. There was no internal evidence of blunt force-penetrating injury to the thoraco-abdominal region. The heart weighed 487 g and there was focal atherosclerosis and 70% stenosis in the mid portion of the left anterior descending artery. The right lung weighed 1089 g and the left lung weighed 1090 g. No focal lesions were noted. The liver weighed 2225 g and the brain weighed 1480 g. The skull showed no evidence of injury or abnormality. The neck showed no evidence of trauma and the hyoid bone and larynx were intact. The medical examiner ruled the death an accident. He also concluded that the detainee died of hypoxic encephalopathy and complications caused by asphyxia and aspiration of stomach contents during restraint. Manic-depressive psychosis was contributory.

## Case 12

A homeless schizophrenic detainee was being booked into jail for attempting to enter a day-care school. He was standing at the booking counter with his hands handcuffed behind his back. He refused to answer intake questions and kicked the sergeant in the head, splitting his ear. Three officers took him to the floor and secured his legs with leg irons. They attempted to place him in a restraint chair but were unsuccessful as he violently struggled with the officers. They carried him to a cell, removed his leg irons, and attempted to restrain with a "kick-stop" restraint strap. The detainee continued to kick and thrash in the cell and the strap broke. The officers secured him with leg irons and additional handcuffs, and placed him in a maximum restrained position. They instituted a 15-minute watch and returned to the cell within 12 minutes. They found the detainee unresponsive, began CPR, and summoned paramedics. Life-saving efforts were unsuccessful.

The decedent was 41 years old, measured 70 inches tall, and weighed 275 pounds. He had a 28-year history of mental illness, having been hospitalized 30 times in a VA hospital. He had been abusing cocaine and alcohol, and had not been taking his prescribed medication for about 9 days. The autopsy showed that he had minor injuries (abrasions and contusions) associated with the struggle with officers, not contributory to his death. There were no injuries to the neck or head and there were no brain abnormalities. His heart weight 491 g and moderate focal coronary arterial atherosclerosis was noted. No abnormalities were noted in the liver, spleen, kidneys, or lungs. A toxicology report noted an absence of any chemicals. The pathologist classified the manner of death as accidental. Contributing factors were cardiac dysrhythmia, postural asphyxia, and acute manic exhaustion. The pathologist further concluded that the intense physical activity with associated high heart rate, catecholamine release, and physiological oxygen debt increased his susceptibility to hypoxia.

## Detention Deaths Due to a Chemical Substance

Detention officers have also experienced sudden restraint custodial deaths of detainees who were under the influence of a chemical substance, as the following example illustrates.

## Case 13

On a traffic stop, a motorist was observed to swallow a gray substance as the officer approached the car. He struggled with the two responding officers and they handcuffed him. He informed the officers that he swallowed a marijuana joint laced with cocaine. He was offered medical care and declined several times. He was brought before the magistrate 30 minutes later exhibiting no medical distress. He was lodged at the jail and did not complain of any medical problems at the time of intake. He was placed into a cell and 45 minutes later, on a second security check, he was found to be unresponsive. Advanced cardiac life support was administered and he was transported by medical personnel to the hospital, where he died 30 minutes later.

The decedent was a 39-year-old African-American male who was 6 feet tall and weighed 195 pounds. He had a history of chronic cocaine, alcohol, and marijuana abuse. The autopsy showed that he did not incur any acute external

**Table 4**
**Location of Death and Time of Incident**

| Location | N | % |
|---|---|---|
| On scene/jail cell | 87 | 60 |
| During transport by police | 30 | 20 |
| Hospital | 14 | 10 |
| During transport by EMS | 14 | 10 |
| Time of Incident | | |
| 12 am to 11:59 am | 55 | 38 |
| 12 pm to 11:59 pm | 90 | 62 |

or internal injuries. He had a rectal temperature of 104°F degrees. His heart was enlarged, weighing 478 g with no gross coronary artery disease. There were apparent lesions in the left ventricle consistent of apparent infiltration in areas of interstitial hemorrhage with wavy fibers consistent with previous ischemia. The left chest cavity contained approx 100 mL of sanguineous fluid with approx 10 mL of similar fluid present in the abdominal cavity. There were no hemorrhages or contusions to the neck. The pulmonary vessels were unremarkable and the distal airways contain edema fluid. The skull was intact and unremarkable and examination of the brain showed no abnormalities. Other organs were found to be unremarkable. The right lung weighed 760 g, the left lung weighed 780 g, the liver weighed 1336 g, the spleen weighed 113 g, and the brain weighed 1244 g. On toxicology, urine analysis revealed cocaine levels of 41 mg/L, benzoylecgonine at 14 mg/L, and for the presence of marijuana. The cause of death was determined to be anoxic encephalopathy as a result of cocaine ingestion. Cardiopulmonary arrest was the result of taking cocaine. Also associated with the cocaine ingestion was rhabdomyolysis and visceral congestion.

As shown in Table 4, 80% of the fatalities in this analysis died on scene or during transport in the police vehicle en route to the jail, police precinct, or hospital. In many jurisdictions, it is customary to transport individuals to the jail or to the precinct in order to determine the condition of the subject and to decide what charges will be lodged. Although these incidents can occur at any time of the day, more than 60% occurred in the afternoon and evening. Moreover, more than 66% occurred during the weekend, Friday evening through Sunday night.

The manner and causes of death are shown in Table 5. The most common manner of death classification was accident (52%). In 23% of cases, the manner was undetermined. The most frequent cause of death identified by the medical examiner or pathologist was acute cocaine or drug toxicity. Physical restraint rendered in police custody was considered contributory in 43% of

**Table 5**
**Manner and Cause of Death in Police Custody (N = 145)**

| Manner of death | N | % |
|---|---|---|
| Accident | 76 | 52 |
| Undetermined | 34 | 23 |
| Natural | 25 | 21 |
| Homicide | 10 | 7 |
| Cause of Death | | |
| Acute cocaine toxicity/drug toxicity, physical restraint in police custody contributory | 62 | 43 |
| Cardiorespiratory arrest associated with psychotic reaction, struggle, and positional restraint | 45 | 31 |
| Positional asphyxiation during restraint for excited delirium | 20 | 14 |
| Acute exhaustive mania during police restraint | 16 | 11 |
| Acute bronchial asthma due to pepper spray and cardiorespiratory arrest | 2 | 1 |

cases. Overall, drug toxicity, cardiorespiratory arrest, or positional asphyxiation during restraint accounted for 88% of the causes of death as attributed by the medical examiner or pathologist on autopsy.

## DISCUSSION

In this case series analysis, a number of common findings emerge. Most cases involved men in their early 30s exhibiting symptomatologies associated with excited delirium. Police are often called to respond to a disturbance/suspicious behavior call (normally misdemeanors), and must utilize mechanical restraints and a variety of other force measures and equipment to control the violent individual. A majority (80%) of the arrestees died in police custody (e.g., on scene or during transport), and the cause of death (43%) was the result of acute cocaine or drug toxicity (drug combinations are common), with physical restraint in police custody suggested as a contributory cause by the medical examiner.

Although detention officers may confront a detainee who is under the influence of a recreational drug, they often encounter a mentally impaired detainee who violently resists physical control and restraint. Police and detention officers are more likely to use empty-hand control techniques, pepper spray, handcuffs, and leg restraints. As tasers are being adopted in more police agencies, it is likely that their use in these types of incidents will increase.

A sudden death in police custody after a force altercation will generally raise a number of questions by the media, the public, the medico-legal investigator, as well as police administrative personnel. The primary questions normally focus on who is responsible for the death and the cause and manner of death. In-custody deaths can place the pathologist and police personnel in a precarious position and there are no easy answers to these types of questions. Because there may be many factors that contribute to an in-custody sudden death, reliance on one factor may be problematic. Several conditions exist that may be associated with sudden death, where no significant pathology is found, such as stress-/fright-related cardiac rhythm disturbances, coronary artery spasm, heart disease, drug toxicity, and neuroleptic malignant syndrome.

As evidenced by this research and the 13 case examples presented here, there are common components that underscore these incidents. First, all of the subjects exhibited bizarre and violent behavior indicative of excited delirium. Second, a majority of the decedents whom the police encountered were under the influence of recreational drugs (69%). Death can occur with both excited delirium, as well as drug or cocaine toxicity (particularly combinations of drugs such as cocaethylene). It should be recognized that in many cases of excited delirium, deaths occur without significant police restraint.

Third, a cardiac condition, particularly an enlarged heart, was a significant risk factor associated with custodial deaths. The mean heart weight of these decedents was 425 g. Diseased or enlarged hearts can be susceptible to sudden dysrhythmias when under physiological stress as occurs with violent struggle, drug toxicity, alcohol, and exhibited abnormal psychological states. Furthermore, psychological stress can induce fatal cardiac arrhythmias, particularly with vulnerable heart condition.

Fourth, 31% of these deaths involved a person who had a history of mental illness, primarily a bipolar disease known as manic-depressive or schizophrenia. Possible factors associated with these deaths are restraint stress, acute psychosis, acute exhaustive mania, the influence of a drugs, noncompliance with psychiatric medications, and underlying cardiac conditions. Individuals suffering from mental illness who are enraged are more susceptible to acute exhaustive mania or neuroleptic malignant syndrome, and those individuals who are/or have a history of abusing various drugs appear to be more at risk to an unexpected death in custody than other individuals.

Fifth, pathologists have included the theory of positional asphyxia as a cause of death in some of these cases in the past *(31,32)*, particularly when the subject is maximally restrained and placed in a prone position (commonly referred as "hogtied"). A positional asphyxiation death owing to being placed in the hogtied position was premised on a former theory attempting to explain deaths after police restraint. This theory has been refuted in several research studies, Chan et al. *(33–36)* and Schmidt et al. *(37)*. These studies found no evidence of hypoxia, hypercapnia, or delay in heart recovery in research subjects while in the restraint position after exercise. Although these studies reveal that hogtying is physiological neutral in regard to positional asphyxiation. It is unknown whether other factors, such as excited delirium *(38,39)*, alcohol/drug intoxication *(20,39)*, trauma from the struggle, hyperactivity, or physiologic stress (*see* Chapter 5, this volume), may be associated with an increase in the susceptibility for sudden death.

The causes and contributory factors of these custodial deaths are varied and complex. Although there are numerous factors that must be considered prior to determining the cause or contributing elements of death, this research suggests there is strong evidence that drug abuse, components of psychosis, and the condition of the internal organs, particularly the heart, play significant roles in an unexpected custodial death. A detailed investigation must be performed and a thorough autopsy must be conducted that analyzes the totality of person's history and the incident facts. In determining the cause and manner of death, the medical examiner is encouraged to analyze all of the circumstantial data, forensic information, and all other available information objectively. It is critical to completely review all the reports of events surrounding the death *(1)*. It is also important to take into account the circumstances of death, environment at the scene, social and medical history, autopsy findings, and toxicological results *(1)*. Police and correctional officers should not be so concerned with labels or classification, but rather with behaviors of the person, and the psychological nature of the confrontation when deciding what measures to use in physically controlling the person.

## REFERENCES

1. Luke JL, Reay DT. The perils of investigating and certifying deaths in police custody. Am J Forensic Med Pathol 1992;13:98–100.
2. Chan TC, Neuman T, Clausen J, Eisele J, Vilke GM. Weight force during prone restraint and respiratory function. Am J Forensic Med Pathol 2004;3:185–189.
3. Reay DT, Howard JD, Flinger CL, Ward RJ. 1988; Effects of positional restraint an oxygen saturation and heart rate following exercise. Am J Forensic Med Pathol 1988;9:16–18.
4. Reay DT, Flinger CL, Stillwell AD, Arnold J. Positional asphyxiation during law enforcement transport. Am J Forensic Med Pathol 1992;13:10–14.
5. O'Halloran RL, Lewman LV. Restraint asphyxiation in excited delirium. Am J Forensic Med Pathol 1993;114:289–285.
6. Wetli CV, Fishbain DA. Cocaine-induced psychosis and sudden death in recreational cocaine users. J Forensic Sci 1985;30:873–880.

7. Mittleman RE, Wetli CV. Cocaine and sudden "natural" death. J Forensic Sci 1987;32:9–11.
8. Wetli CV. Fatal cocaine intoxication. Am J Forensic Med Pathol 1987;8:1–2.
9. Baker FM. Cocaine psychosis. J Natl Med Assoc 1987;81:992–1000.
10. Kosten TR, Kleber HD. Rapid death during cocaine abuse: a variant of the neuroleptic malignant syndrome? Am J Drug Alcohol Abuse 1988;14:335–346.
11. Wetli CV, Mash D, Karch SB. Cocaine-associated agitated delirium and the neuroleptic malignant syndrome. Am J Emerg Med 1996;14:425–428.
12. McLaughlin V, Siddle BK. Law enforcement custody deaths. Police Chief 1988;8:38–41.
13. Kornblum RN, Reddy SK. Effects of taser in fatalities involving police confrontation. J Forensic Sci 1991;36:343–348.
14. Krosh C, Binkard V, Blackbourn B. Final report of custody task force, San Diego Police Department, San Diego, CA, 1992.
15. Mirchandani HG, Rorke LB, Sekula-Perlman A, Hood IC. Cocaine-induced agitated delirium, forceful struggle, and minor head injury. Am J Forensic Med Pathol 1994;15:95–99.
16. Granfield J, Kami O, Petty C. Pepper spray and in-custody deaths. Science and Technology, International Associations of Chiefs of Police, Alexandria, VA, 1994, pp. 1–5.
17. Pollanen MS, Chiasson DA, Cairns JT, Young JG. Unexpected death related to restraint for excited delirium: A retrospective study of deaths in police custody and the community. Can Med Assoc J 1998;12:1603–1607.
18. Ross DL. Factors associated with excited delirium deaths in police custody. Mod Pathol 1998;11:1127–1137.
19. O'Halloran RL, Frank JG. Asphyxial death during prone restraint revisited: A report of 21 cases. Am J Forensic Med Pathol 2000;21:39–52.
20. Stratton SJ, Rogers C, Green K. Sudden death in individuals on hobble restraint during paramedic transport. Ann Emerg Med 1995;25:170–712.
21. Spitz WU. Capture myopathy. JAMA 1985;43:253.
22. Lown B. Sudden cardiac death: bio-behavioral perspective. Circulation 1987;76 (Suppl.):186–189.
23. Engel GL. Sudden and rapid death during psychological stress. Ann Internal Med 1971;74:771–782.
24. Cebelin MS, Hirsch CS. Human stress cardiomyopathy. Hum Pathol 1980;11:123–132.
25. Ruttenber AJ, Lawler-Heavner J, Ming Y, Wetli CV, Hearn WL, Mash DC. Fatal excited delirium following cocaine use: epidemiologic findings provide new evidence for mechanisms of cocaine toxicity. J Forensic Sci 1997;42:25–31.
26. Krosch C. Some in-custody deaths cited as preventable. Law Enforcement Q 1992;4:15–18, 35.
27. Lapasota EA. Cocaine-induced heart disease: mechanisms and pathology. J Thorac Imaging 1991;6:68–75.
28. Post RB. Cocaine psychosis: a continuum model. Am J Psychiatry 1975;32:225–230.

29. Bunn WH, Giannini AJ. Cardiovascular complications of cocaine abuse. Am Fam Physician 1992;46:769–777.

30. Essobedo LG, Ruttenber JA, Agoes M, Anda RR, Wetli CV. Emerging patterns of cocaine use and epidemic of cocaine overdose, deaths in Dade County Florida. Arch Pathol Lab Med 1992;115:900–905.

31. Reay DT. Suspect restraint and sudden death. FBI Law Enforcement Bulletin 1996;May:22–25.

32. Bell MD, Rao VJ, Wetli CV. Positional asphyxiation in adults. Am J Forensic Med Pathol 1992;13:25–28.

33. Chan TC, Vilke GM, Neuman T, Clausen JL. Restraint position and positional asphyxia. Ann Emerg Med 1997;30:578–586.

34. Chan TC, Vilke GM, Neuman T. Reexamination of custody restraint position and positional asphyxia. Am J Forensic Med Pathol 1998;19:201–205.

35. Chan TC, Vilke GM, Clausen J, et al. The effect of oleoresin capsicum pepper spray inhalation on respiratory function. J Forensic Sci 2002;47:299–304.

36. Chan T.C, Vilke G.M, Clausen J, et al. Pepper spray's effects on a suspect's ability to breathe. National Institute of Justice: Research in Brief, U.S. Department of Justice, Washington, DC, 2001, pp. 1–7.

37. Schmidt P, Snowden T. The effects of positional restraint on heart rate and oxygen saturation. J Emerg Med 1999;5:777–782.

38. Karch S, Wetli CV. Agitated delirium versus positional asphyxiation. American Medical Care, New York, NY, 1995, pp. 760–761.

39. Giles GH, Sandrin S. Alcohol deaths in police custody. Alcohol Clin Exp Res 1992; 32:419–432.

# Chapter 10

# Deaths in Custody Investigations

*Vincent Di Miao*

The death of an individual at the time of arrest or in police custody has the potential for generation of civil litigation, criminal charges against law enforcement personnel, and, on occasion, riots. Some segments of our society are distrustful of police. On occasion, this distrust is justified. In most instances, however, there is no misconduct. The situation is often aggravated by the news media, which seems sensation-driven. Thorough investigation and thoughtful analysis of an incident is often lacking.

The public and the media look for simple answers to complex problems. They often confuse proximity of an action with causality, an error in logic identified by Aristotle more than 2300 years ago. If an investigation into the death does not satisfy their initial assumptions, they often claim conspiracy or "cover-up."

In-custody deaths fall into three categories, temporally: those occurring at the time of arrest, those while being transported to jail or a hospital, and those while the deceased is a resident of the jail. The causes of death may be a natural disease, accidental trauma, suicide, homicidal trauma, or the sequelae of a cascade of natural physiological reactions to stress, often aggravated by drugs. No matter how the case presents, it is always best to treat all cases as if one is dealing with a homicide in which there will be subsequent judicial proceedings. It is always better to do too much in such cases than too little.

The medico-legal investigation of an in-custody death should ideally have three components: the investigation, the autopsy, and subsequent laboratory tests.

From: *Forensic Science and Medicine: Sudden Deaths in Custody*
Edited by: D. L. Ross and T. C. Chan © Humana Press Inc., Totowa, NJ

## THE INVESTIGATION

The following steps should be taken as part of the investigation:

1. The scene of the death should be visited and documented photographically. Diagrams may be made if it is felt that they may be of aid.
2. A complete account of the circumstances surrounding the fatal incident should be obtained. The actions of individuals involved immediately prior to, at and after the death should be determined. Police reports of the incident, including copies of interviews with the police officers involved, witnesses, and medical personnel should be obtained.
3. Medical records of the fatal incident should be obtained. It should be determined if and when any drugs were administered or medical procedures conducted.
4. Past medical records of the deceased should be obtained.
5. If the deceased was on any medications, this information should be determined. One should determine the dosage taken, the frequency taken, and how long the individual was on the medication.
6. The results of any police laboratory examinations should be obtained.
7. If the individual was hospitalized, any blood taken on admission to the hospital should be sought and obtained.

The material included in this list is then submitted to the office where a detailed report is prepared for the forensic pathologist who will be performing the autopsy. The material should be retained for subsequent closer review by the forensic pathologist. Some of the information (e.g., interviews) may not be initially available. The investigation report may be supplemented by information subsequently obtained from additional witnesses, other agencies, police reports, and crime lab reports.

## THE AUTOPSY

A complete autopsy should be conducted. The autopsy should be performed by or under the direct supervision of an experienced forensic pathologist, board certified in anatomical and p by the American Board of Pathology. The autopsy should include a detailed examination of the external aspects of the body for evidence of disease or trauma. Any trauma noted should be specifically located on the body, described in detail, measured, and photographed. The deceased's clothing should also be examined for evidence of violence. Photographs of the body should be taken even in the absence of injuries to document the absence.

The internal examination of the body should include examination of all three body cavities (i.e., the cranial cavity, the thoracic, and the abdomen). The neck organs should be removed and examined in detail. When felt necessary by the pathologist, additional incisions and examinations should be made. Any trauma noted should be described in detail, measured, and photographed. A microscopic survey of all organs, especially the heart, should be performed. Body fluids should be retained for toxicological analysis.

## LABORATORY TESTING

In all cases, a complete toxicological screen should be performed. In special circumstances, one may want to retain the brain for subsequent examination by a neuropathologist. Genetic testing may be considered if one suspects an entity such as the prolonged QT syndrome.

In all cases, it is recommended that at the minimum, blood, vitreous, urine, and bile be obtained for toxicological analysis. All specimens should be collected with a clean needle and a new syringe. The specimens should be placed in glass containers, not plastic as these fluids can leach out plastic polymers from the wall of a plastic container. On subsequent examination, by gas chromatography (GC), the polymers may interfere with analysis. Collect at a minimum 50 mL of blood. Place 20 mL in a 20-mL red-top glass test tube; 20 mL in two 10-mL gray-top glass test tubes (preservative potassium oxalate and sodium fluoride), and 10 mL in a purple-top glass test tube (preservative EDTA). Collect all the vitreous; 20 mL of urine and up to 20 mL of bile. Label the specimens as to name of deceased; case number; date of examination; name of the pathologist and, in the case of the blood, the source of the blood. If the blood is to be analyzed for volatiles, then some of it should be kept in a test tube with a Teflon-lined screw top.

Blood should be collected from the femoral or subclavian vessels to prevent the possibility of postmortem release (redistribution) of drugs from tissue into blood, with resultant artifactually elevated blood levels.

In individuals who have died in the hospital, any drugs in the blood at the time of admission may have been metabolized. The hospital in which the individual was a patient should be contacted to see if any blood obtained at or shortly after hospitalization is still in existence. This should then be obtained for toxicological analysis.

The urine is generally of use only in screening for drugs as detection only indicates that the individual has taken that drug at some time in the past, not that he or she is under the influence of it. It is the presence of the drug in the blood that is of importance.

After blood, vitreous humor is next in value. Virtually any drug detectable in the blood is detectable in the vitreous if one uses analytical techniques and equipment of sufficient sensitivity. With the exception of alcohol, the significance of the level present is another matter.

Analysis of specimen may be conducted by GC, gas chromatography mass spectrometry (GC-MS), high-performance liquid chromatography, immunoassay, or ultraviolet spectrophotometry. It must be realized that except for GC-MS, none of the methods is totally specific. All that the other analytical methods provide is presumptive evidence of the presence of the drug. Although the presumptive evidence may be very strong, another testing procedure must be performed for positive identification. The confirmatory test must involve a totally different method of analysis from the one originally used. If initial analysis is made with the GC-MS, there is no need to redo the identification because this method is specific.

Specimens for toxicological analysis should be retained for 5 years.

## MICROSCOPY

At the time of autopsy, tissue should be retained from all the major organs for microscopic examination. At least six sections of heart should be examined with at least one coming from the area of the conduction system. All microscopic slides and paraffin blocks should be retained indefinitely. Tissue removed at autopsy should be retained for 5 years.

## CERTIFICATION OF DEATH

Following the autopsy, if there is no evidence of sufficient trauma to explain death, this information should be released to the public. No ruling as to the cause of death should be made until all the investigation and testing is complete.

Two of the most important functions of a forensic pathologist are the determination of the cause and manner of death. The *cause of death* is any injury or disease that produces a physiological derangement in the body that results in the individual dying. Examples of causes of death are a gunshot wound, a stab wound of the chest, adenocarcinoma of the lung, or coronary atherosclerosis. *The mechanism of death* is the physiological derangement produced by the cause of death that results in death. Examples of mechanism of death would be hemorrhage, septicemia, and cardiac arrhythmia.

*The manner of death* explains how the cause of death came about. The manners of death are natural, homicide, suicide, accident, and undetermined. The manner of death is an opinion based on the known facts concerning the circumstances leading up to and surrounding the death in conjunction with the findings at autopsy and the laboratory tests. A manner of death is ruled undetermined when there is insufficient information about the circumstances surrounding the death to make a ruling, or when the cause of death is unknown.

Occasionally, there are cases in which the cause of death would ordinarily be considered natural, but the manner is homicide. Thus, we have the home-owner who surprises the burglar, engaging him in a violent struggle only to collapse and die of a heart attack. The mechanism of death is a cardiac arrhythmia and the cause of death is severe coronary atherosclerosis, but the manner of death is homicide in that the arrhythmia was brought on or precipitated by the struggle.

Certification as to the cause of death in deaths occurring in police custody may vary from simple to extremely complex. In a case of suicide by hanging in a jail, if one has excluded intervention by others and performed a complete autopsy, the cause of death can be certified as "asphyxia by hanging" with the manner of death suicide. If death is the result of obvious injury such as a skull fracture, then one must attempt to determine whether the injury predates the arrest. If it does not, then it must be determined whether it occurred during the arrest procedure or while in jail. In the latter case, it needs to be determined whether death was a result of a fall or an attack by another inmate or police. If it were the result of a fall as determined by autopsy, then the case would be an accident. If the deceased was knocked or thrown to the ground, the case is a homicide. If the injury is owing to a blow, it is a homicide, no matter who inflicted the injury. Natural deaths can be readily assigned to their cause and the manner natural.

The problem arises in deaths occurring during episodes of excited delirium. If the case is truly caused by positional asphyxia (e.g., placing an obese individual over a transmission hump in a vehicle), then the manner of death is accident. If it is owing to positional asphyxia because officers are inappropriately holding a person down, then it is a homicide.

If death results from the cascade of physiological changes that produces death as in most cases of excited delirium, local custom may reign as to ascribing the cause and manner of death. There are two common ways of signing out such cases. First is to sign out the cause of death as "excited delirium" and then list "struggle," "cocaine intoxication," and so on, as contributory causes. The other way is to sign out the cause of death in a descriptive manner (e.g., "Cardiopulmonary arrest during violent struggle in individual under influence of cocaine, alcohol, etc."). In individuals with psychoses, this is listed either as a contributory cause or incorporated in the descriptive diagnosis. The greater difficulty is designating a manner of death. Because of the effects of the violent struggle, one cannot classify such a case as a natural death. One is then left with homicide or accident. Because a violent struggle has occurred with interaction between two or more individuals, the best classification of the manner of death is probably homicide. A good argument for an accident can be made, however.

If the case is called a homicide, one must explain to questioners that the designation of the case as a homicide does not indicate that there was necessarily any criminal activity involved. The difference between homicide and murder should be carefully explained.

When the cause and manner of death are determined, this information should be released by the medico-legal agency and not the police agency involved. Some police agencies like to have a joint press conference with the forensic pathologist who made the ruling when the announcement is made. This is undesirable. The reason that the cause and manner of death should be released exclusively by the medico-legal office is to prevent the appearance of collusion with the police agency.

## REFERENCE

1. Di Maio VJM, Di Maio DJ. Forensic pathology 2nd ed. CRC Press, Boca Raton, FL, 2001.

# Chapter 11

# Liability and Wrongful In-Custody Deaths

*Darrell L. Ross*

Sudden deaths in police or correctional custody after a use-of-force confrontation are emerging as a critical area in civil litigation. This chapter describes the potential civil liability issues commonly associated with wrongful custodial deaths involving deaths following restraint incidents. Liability issues involving standards of care in state courts are examined, as well as the standards for use of force, restraints, and medical care in accordance with actions stemming from claims of negligence and Section 1983. Although many of these lawsuits are settled out of court, those cases that are decided in court yield a number of essential legal issues worthy of concern for police officers and administrators. Custodial deaths normally will produce a civil lawsuit by the estate attempting to demonstrate that the officers and governmental entity should be held responsible for a wrongful death.

## PLAINTIFF ASSERTIONS OF WRONGFUL CUSTODIAL DEATHS

A lawsuit filed in a wrongful custodial death will allege that the agency as a whole was intentionally negligent, grossly negligent, and deliberately indifferent to the needs of the deceased. The lawsuit generally will assert that the department's custom, policy, and procedures (or lack thereof) were the "proximate cause" of the death.

The claim may also assert that the department fails to keep abreast of changes in the profession, and that it takes a death or a lawsuit before the agency makes necessary changes. Generally, the following allegations are made

From: *Forensic Science and Medicine: Sudden Deaths in Custody*
Edited by: D. L. Ross and T. C. Chan © Humana Press Inc., Totowa, NJ

against public officials in a sudden wrongful death (not mutually exclusive): excessive force used by the arresting officers, officers assaulted and battered the deceased, the officers' use of restraints or force methods contributed to the decedent's death, the officers were grossly negligent or deliberately indifferent to the medical and/or psychological needs of the deceased, officers failed to assess/monitor the medical condition or to provide/summon medical assistance for the deceased, officers failed to transport the deceased to the nearest hospital or summon medical assistance at the arrest scene, the officers failed to follow departmental policy, the decedent in a maximum restrained position was transported in a police vehicle, which contributed to his or her death, officers violated the decedent's constitutional rights, officers acted outside the scope of their authority, and officers conspired to injure or cause the death of the deceased.

The claim may also assert that administrative personnel failed to provide officers with policies that would direct them in responding to "special needs" arrestees (drug-induced or mentally impaired), failed to provide officers with training in how to properly respond and use force-control techniques with special needs arrestees, failed to provide officers with appropriate equipment to perform their duties, failed to supervise their officers, failed to train supervisors, negligently entrusted equipment to their officers without training or competency evaluation, condoned excessive force measures with arrestees, failed to articulate directives in how to transport special needs arrestees, failed to develop protocols for responding to violent arrestee's medical/psychological needs, conspired to cause the death of the deceased, failed to conduct an internal or independent investigation of the death, and covered up the death with a less than adequate investigation. Each case will obviously comprise numerous variables for the plaintiff to attack. In any lawsuit, not all initial allegations will withstand judicial scrutiny. The agency should, however, be prepared to justify and defend each claim.

## Negligence Components

The common law and statutes generally provide that the police may take custody of the apparently mentally ill or those who appear to be dangerous *(1)*. Negligence claims against police officers for wrongful deaths of arrestees are based on state tort law. Negligence tort definitions differ from state to state, and are generally differentiated from other torts as it includes inadvertent behavior that results in injury or damage *(2)*. In some states, slight negligence will suffice, whereas other states require gross negligence, which involves a reckless disregard of the consequences of behaviors. When an arrestee dies in police custody, a presumption of negligence may arise, if the arresting officers failed to follow departmental policies regarding force measures, use of restraints, medical concerns, and transporting procedures.

Wrongful death torts, usually established by law and found in all states, arise whenever a death occurs as a result of an officer's unjustified action *(3)*. These lawsuits are based on state statutes and brought by the estate of the deceased *(4)*. Frequently, wrongful death claims emerge from a deadly force incident, however, deaths in custody after a physical force altercation and custodial suicides have become the subject of more wrongful death litigation. The possibility of a wrongful death lawsuit arises any time a death is caused by the criminal justice personnel, however, no liability attaches unless the death was unjustified *(5)*. Furthermore, the claim must be based on a recognized tort theory. Compensatory and punitive damages can be awarded.

The standard applied in negligence torts is whether the officer's act or failure to act created an unreasonable risk to another individual. When police officers exercise custodial control over a person, they have a duty to provide reasonable care (*Thomas v. Williams,* 1962; *Wagar v. Hasenkrug,* 1980; *Abraham v. Maes,* 1983). Custody applies to police arresting/transporting or detention officers confining prisoners and the mentally impaired. This means that the police have a legal duty to take reasonable precautions to ensure the health and safety of persons in their custody, render medical assistance as warranted, and treat arrestees humanely. Establishing negligence is difficult. Four components must be established to prove a negligence claim: legal duty, breach of duty, proximate cause of injury, and actual injury.

A legal duty requires an officer either to act or refrain from acting in particular situations. They may arise from laws, customs, judicial decisions, and various agency regulations *(6)*. Once the plaintiff has proved a duty, it must be demonstrated that the officer breached the duty by failing to act in accordance with the legal responsibility. Courts recognize that the police are only liable to specific individuals and not to the general public. There must exist some special knowledge or circumstances that sets the individual citizen apart from the general public and shows a relationship between that citizen and the police *(4)*. Next, if the plaintiff can show that the officer owed a duty, and breached that duty, it must be established that the officer was the proximate cause for the harm or the damage *(2)*. A close causal link between the officer's negligent conduct and the consequent harm to the arrestee must be proven. To maintain liability it must be proven that actual damage or injury was incurred as a result of the officer's negligent conduct.

These components provide the structure in which a state tort claim for negligence in a wrongful custodial death will be examined. Many courts define proximate cause. It may be enough to show that the officer's behavior or omission to act rose to a level that caused the injury or death of the arrestee. Although other courts may rely on a higher standard of recklessness, wanton conduct or gross negligence before negligence will be attached. For example in *Tindall v. Multnomah County* (1977), there was no negligence when an officer took the intoxicated decedent to jail rather than to a treatment facility after being notified by hospital personnel that they would not take drunks. The officer did not inform detention personnel that the arrestee had fallen and had a bump on his head. There was no violation of a state statute because the statute was applicable only when the arrestee was incapacitated or in immediate danger, and if a treatment facility was available. A cause for liability was upheld in *Brinkman v. City of Indianapolis* (1967), however, when an officer took a severely sick man to jail rather than to a hospital, provided no medical assistance, and notified the man's relatives that they could not post bond until the morning.

## Special Duty of Care

Courts have also established that an officer may owe a special duty when there is reason to believe that the arrestee presents a danger to him or herself. When it is evident that a particular arrestee has a diminished ability or cannot exercise the same level of care as an ordinary person because of mental illness or intoxication, police must ensure that reasonable measures are taken in order to care for the person in their custody (*Thomas v. Williams,* 1962; *Shuff v. Zurich*, 1965).

The concept of special duty is based on two factors: (a) officer's knowledge of the arrestee's mental state, and (b) the extent in which the condition renders the arrestee unable to exercise ordinary care. If it is foreseeable (a reasonable anticipation that the injury or damage is likely as a result of an act or omission) that a circumstance shows an arrestee's condition creates a hazard, a general duty of care is required of police and transferred into a special duty of care that may lead to liability if the duty is beached. If an officer possesses sufficient knowledge of an arrestee's mental or intoxicated condition and the arrestee is rendered helpless, a special duty to render care may exist.

A special duty of care creates higher responsibilities and may include cases of unexpected custodial deaths. In *Fruge v. City of New Orleans* (1993) the estate brought a wrongful death claim for a diabetic arrestee who gave an appearance of intoxication. An arrestee was placed in an isolation cell, where he later was observed to be foaming at the mouth. He was transported to the hospital and died 2 hours later. The attending doctor stated that the arrestee had a moderately enlarged liver, which can cause sudden death. The court found that officers were negligent in their decision to incarcerate the man as they owed a duty to the prisoner to protect him from harm and preserve his safety. The court concluded that the city failed in its responsibility (duty breached) by not ascertaining the man's medical condition and transporting him to a hospital. The arrestee's intoxication triggered the need for a higher degree of care by the police.

In *Del Tufo v. Township of Old Bridge* (1996), the estate of an arrestee, who died from cocaine overdose while in police custody, brought a wrongful death action for negligence. The estate claimed that officers failed to provide emergency medical assistance upon arrest. Officers responded to a traffic accident and found the driver (decedent) sitting at the wheel with the motor running. Officers attempted to subdue and restrain the arrestee, but he violently struggled with them. Other officers responded and he was restrained with his hands behind his back and placed in the backseat of the patrol car. In the patrol car, he began kicking the windows and during transport the officer observed him to be shaking violently. At police headquarters the arrestee collapsed outside the car. The officer removed the handcuffs, initiated cardiopulmonary resuscitation (CPR), and called for medical assistance. The individual died 1 hour later at the hospital from cardiac failure due to ingesting 1.5 to 3.5 g of cocaine.

The court acknowledged that the police have a duty to provide emergency medical assistance to those in their custody. However, the court rejected the idea that drug abusers fall into the same category as the elderly and the mentally ill, as they have a responsibility to advise the police that they have consumed drugs—self-inflicted harm equates to self-care responsibility. The plaintiff failed to prove that the officers were the proximate cause of the death of the arrestee by a delay of medical care and comparative fault was used as the defense for the officers: "a policy of individual responsibility for voluntary behavior."

The estate in *Brown v. Lee* (1994) brought a wrongful death claim when the deceased died in the police lockup from an overdose of methylenedioxymethamphetamine (e.g., Ecstasy). The plaintiff asserted that the sheriff had a duty to obtain medical treatment for him. The lawsuit alleged negligent failure to provide medical care and negligence in monitoring arrestees in the lockup. The deceased was arrested on charges of disturbing the peace because he was walking in the middle of traffic, sweating, and grimacing. The arresting officer detected the odor of alcohol and during transport asked him if he had used the drug Ecstasy. He denied any drug use, although he acted "hyper" and was sweating. The arrestee said he was fine during booking. Medical attention was offered but he refused and was placed in a cell.

During the night, a trustee noticed that the decedent was experiencing breathing difficulties and shaking, and the trustee called for the officers. Responding officers found the arrestee dead. An autopsy revealed that he died from a drug overdose. The court acknowledged that officers owed a duty to provide care for arrestees and a higher degree of care is owed to an intoxicated person who cannot care for him or herself. Because the arrestee denied being under the influence and denied medical care when offered and because the drug condition is not frequently fatal, the court dismissed the claim stating that it is "unreasonable to impose a duty on the sheriff to provide medical treatment to every intoxicated arrestee."

These cases illustrate that the courts determine a special duty on a case-by-case-basis. The courts expect the police to provide a level of care and caution when taking custody of arrestees who exhibit signs of intoxication and mental illness. Although a plaintiff may be able to prove that an officer owed a duty and breached the duty, he or she must next prove that the officer was the proximate cause of the injury or death. This is not a simple endeavor as there are considerable differences between the court's interpretation of proximate cause. In these unexpected death cases, one method of determining this is to ask whether the arrestee would have died without the officer's action . To determine the true cause of death, careful consideration must be given to the decedent's medical and psychological history and his or her condition hours prior to and during the arrest. In some incidents, the officer's action or inaction may be a significant factor and may rise to a level of culpability resulting in liability. The courts will determine the degree of knowledge the police had at the time or obtained relative to the arrestee's condition in regard to condition and resultant death.

Although a definitive test for foreseeability does not exist, the courts will rely on the individual facts of the circumstances and on existing precedent when analyzing the case. Figure 1 illustrates how the courts determine liability based on negligence factors, special duty, and knowledge/foreseeable factors concerning sudden/wrongful in-custody deaths. Many courts will evaluate the case based on the totality of circumstances. However, other courts will consider the knowledge that the officers possessed about the arrestee who exhibited symptoms associated with sudden deaths and whether the death was foreseeable. The interaction between judicial decision making and factual circumstances that indicate a breach of duty ultimately determines liability for negligent failure to prevent a wrongful death (7).

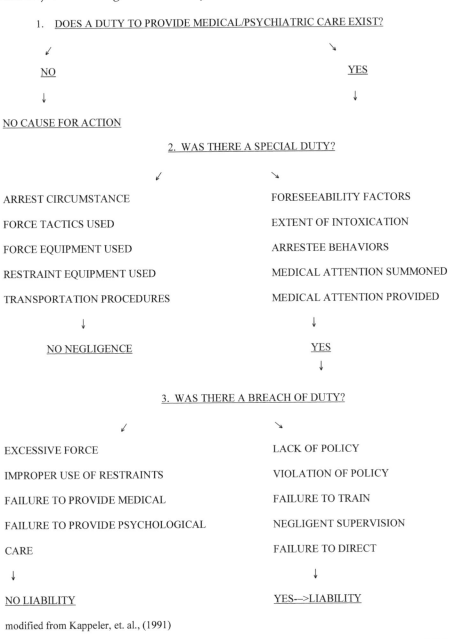

1.  DOES A DUTY TO PROVIDE MEDICAL/PSYCHIATRIC CARE EXIST?

NO                                                                    YES

NO CAUSE FOR ACTION

2.  WAS THERE A SPECIAL DUTY?

ARREST CIRCUMSTANCE                      FORESEEABILITY FACTORS

FORCE TACTICS USED                           EXTENT OF INTOXICATION

FORCE EQUIPMENT USED                     ARRESTEE BEHAVIORS

RESTRAINT EQUIPMENT USED             MEDICAL ATTENTION SUMMONED

TRANSPORTATION PROCEDURES         MEDICAL ATTENTION PROVIDED

NO NEGLIGENCE                                     YES

3.  WAS THERE A BREACH OF DUTY?

EXCESSIVE FORCE                                 LACK OF POLICY

IMPROPER USE OF RESTRAINTS           VIOLATION OF POLICY

FAILURE TO PROVIDE MEDICAL           FAILURE TO TRAIN

FAILURE TO PROVIDE PSYCHOLOGICAL   NEGLIGENT SUPERVISION

CARE                                                       FAILURE TO DIRECT

NO LIABILITY                                        YES-->LIABILITY

modified from Kappeler, et. al., (1991)

**Fig. 1.** Liability decision-making model in police custodial deaths.

## Wrongful Custodial Death Claims Under Section 1983

Wrongful death actions are recognized in all states, therefore, such laws may be utilized in a Section 1983 action. Section 1983 authorizes the application of any state remedial law that is consistent with the purposes of Section 1983 to any situation for which federal civil rights laws do not provide appropriate remedy *(1)*. Wrongful death claims may be filed under Section 1983 when the death has resulted from excessive force, failure to attend to medical needs or any other constitutional violation, and the conduct of the defendants were the proximate cause of the death under intentional tort principles (*Wright v. Collins,* 1985).

Unexpected custodial death cases filed under Section 1983 are evaluated within the purview of the Fourth and Fourteenth Amendments, based on the standards of "deliberate indifference," "objective reasonableness," and "shocks the conscience." The status of the person dictates which amendment standard applies. Table 1 summarizes various liability issues, precedent cases, and applicable standards of review when analyzing the various factors of sudden deaths in police custody. Liability concerns regarding citizens arrested, restrained, and who suddenly expire shortly after arrest, are analyzed according to the Fourth Amendment standard of objective reasonable force, and primarily involve issues of excessive force/restraints, failure to train, failure to render medical/psychological care, and policy and customs issues that are alleged to have violated the decedents' constitutional rights. Medical, psychological, and failure to protect concerns are generally examined under the Eighth and the Fourteenth Amendments deliberate indifference standard. Arrestees' behaviors that are consistent with the inability to provide care for themselves, such as the intoxicated or mentally ill, pose a particular dilemma for responding officers.

Depending on the confinement status of a confined prisoner (jail vs prison), unexpected custodial death cases filed under Section 1983 are evaluated within the purview of the Eighth and Fourteenth Amendments. Detainee deaths in detention centers generally are examined in accordance with the standards of "shocks the conscience" (*Johnson v. Glick,* 1973) and "deliberate indifference" (*Estelle v. Gamble,* 1976). The death of a convicted prisoner is assessed in accordance with the Eighth Amendment standard of cruel and unusual punishment (*Hudson v. McMillian,* 1992) and "deliberate indifference" (*Estelle,* 1976). Pertinent issues and common claims in these cases include excessive force, inappropriate use or abuse of restraints, failure to render medical/psychological care, failure to train, supervise, or direct the officers involved in the case, and policy and customs issues that are alleged to have violated the decedents' constitutional rights. Prisoner behaviors that are consistent with the

**Table 1**
**Sudden Deaths in Police Custody Liability Issues Matrix**

| | Arrestee | | |
| --- | --- | --- | --- |
| Issue | Applicable amendment | Precedent cases | Standard of review |
| Use of force and restraints | Fourth | *Graham v. Conner* (1989) *Tennessee v. Garner* (1985) | Objective reasonableness |
| Medical/p | Fourteenth | *Revere v. Mass General Hospital* (1983) | Deliberate indifference |
| Policy/custom | Fourteenth | *Monell v. Dept. of Social Services, NY* (1978) | Deliberate indifference Proximate cause |
| Training | Fourteenth | *City of Canton v. Harris* (1989) | Deliberate indifference |
| | Pre-trial detainees | | |
| Use of force and restraints | Fifth and Fourteenth | *Johnson v. Glick* (1973) *Bell v. Wolfish* (1979) *Rochin v. CA* (1952) | Shocks conscience Due process clause |
| Medical/ psychological | Eighth and Fourteenth | *Estelle v. Gamble* (1976) *Revere v. MA General Hospital* (1983) | Deliberate indifference |
| Failure to protect | Eighth and Fourteenth | *DeShaney v. Winnebago* (1989) *Farmer v. Brennan* (1994) | Deliberate indifference Special relationship |
| Policy/custom | Fourteenth | *Monell v. Dept. of Social Services* (1978) | Deliberate indifference Proximate Cause |
| Training | Fourteenth | *City of Canton v. Harris* (1989) | Deliberate indifference |

inability to provide care for themselves, such as the intoxicated or mentally ill, pose a particular dilemma for responding officers.

## CASE EXAMPLES IN POLICING

### Claims of Excessive Force

A significant number of sudden death restraint incidents involves violent behaviors of an arrestee requiring police to use higher levels of physical control measures and less lethal force equipment or implements. As a result, the primary claims filed against the responding officers are allegations of excessive force that occurred during the arrest, at the station, or in a detention cell.

In *Estate of Phillips v. City of Milwaukee* (1996), officers used force to subdue a large schizophrenic man who was wielding ballpoint pens in each hand. After a lengthy struggle, the man was controlled, handcuffed behind his back, and further restrained with leg restraints. He was on his stomach for 1 minute and suddenly stopped breathing. CPR was initiated and emergency medical personnel responded but they were unable to revive him. The arrestee died 1 day later and the medical examiner determined that restraint was contributory to death. The estate filed a Section 1983 lawsuit for excessive force, denial of medical care, and failure to train. The court held that the officers did not utilize excessive force tactics in controlling the arrestee. Police actions were analyzed based on the totality of circumstances and the resistive behaviors they encountered. Deliberate indifference to the medical needs of the deceased was not established and officers were shielded from liability under qualified immunity. Moreover, the court noted: "police officers facing unpredictable and oftentimes dangerous situations must be free to perform their duties utilizing their training, experience, and judgment with confidence that courts will not scrutinize their discretionary decisions with microscopic detail" (at 831).

In *East v. City of Chicago* (1989), however, the court held that officers used excessive force when East died of a drug overdose in their custody. During a drug raid, the decedent swallowed a packet of cocaine. Approximately 4 hours later in the interrogation room at the station he experienced hallucinations, began yelling, and attempted to hide under a table. Several officers removed him from under the table, kicked him in the head and between his legs, and hit him with a nightstick in an attempt to handcuff him. East told officers he had ingested cocaine, but they ignored him, and responded "you're just afraid to go to jail." He was placed in a cell with another prisoner who later informed police East needed medical attention. At an unknown time, paramedics were summoned, responded, and transported him to the hospital where he later died.

The court cited the *Graham v. Connor* (1989) decision but acknowledged that the arrestee was in custody at the station when force was applied. They ruled that in post-arrest situations when dealing with a pretrial detainee, the Fourteenth Amendment standard of "shocks the conscience" is applicable. The officers were found liable for beating the arrestee, deliberate indifference to his medical needs under *Estelle v. Gamble* (1976), and the city was also liable for failing to train officers in the appropriate use of force.

In cases of sudden death after force measures are utilized, two general questions are commonly asked: "Was the officer's force excessive?" and "Did the amount of force used contribute to the detainee's death?" Answering these questions is not easy.

The standard of review in excessive force claims stemming from a police arrest situation was established in accordance with the Fourth Amendment and the US Supreme Court's decision in *Graham v. Connor* (1989). The Court determined that "objective reasonableness" is the standard of review for all claims involving Fourth Amendment use of force situations. Although there is no precise definition for the test of reasonableness, applying the standard requires careful attention to the facts and circumstances confronting the police, without regard to their underlying intent or motivation. Each case must be evaluated from the perspective of a reasonable officer on the scene based on the severity of crime, the resistance level of the arrestee, threat of safety posed by the arrestee, and whether the circumstances were rapidly evolving.

The courts recognize that use-of-force incidents involve rapid and tense factors and that officers frequently must respond quickly with the understanding that there are numerous variables to consider. Utilizing the objective reasonableness standard the court will determine whether officers used excessive force by evaluating the totality of the circumstances including the unpredictability and danger and violent behavior manifested by the arrestee, and whether force or control tactics used were reasonable or proportionate in light of the resistive behaviors encountered. Objective reasonable and lawful force is force used at the moment it is needed and in response to the arrestee's behavior regardless of the outcome. The *East* case, however, provides an example of excessive force as officers kicked the arrestee in the head and between the legs and then continued to beat him with an impact weapon. After establishing control, officers failed to provide timely medical assistance. In light of the circumstances, these tactics were considered excessive and disproportionate. Failure to follow up with necessary medical care amounted to deliberate indifference.

## Use-of-Restraint Claims

Associated with excessive force allegations, is a second level of claims that often asserts that the police maximally restrained the deceased, which purportedly contributed to his or her death. The assertion is frequently made that the deceased died as a result of "positional, postural, restraint, compressional, or mechanical asphyxia," because he or she was placed in the "hogtied" position. The claim may also assert that the individual died from asphyxia resulting from the weight of the officers on the individual's body for an extended period during control and restraint. These allegations may be further supported by results of an autopsy or independent autopsy conducted by the estate claiming that the method of restraint contributed to asphyxia, which caused death. Moreover, this assertion will attempt to prove excessive force by utilizing restraints without deference to the obvious medical needs of the arrestee.

A federal court found the City of Chicago liable for contributing to the death of an arrestee under the influence of cocaine and phencyclidine in *Animashaun v. O'Donnell* (1994). While restrained and lying face down on the ground, the arrestee began experiencing breathing difficulties. He was transported to the hospital in a maximally restrained position where he was pronounced dead. The estate filed a Section 1983 action claiming that the decedent died from positional asphyxia resulting from the nature of restraint methods used by the police. City officials contended that they were unaware of the relationship between restraining an arrestee in this manner and the occurrence of positional asphyxia. The plaintiff attached a memorandum of a similar death in 1988 regarding this problem and the City deliberately ignored it. The court held that the City was on notice that its officers were responding to recurring situations yet chose to ignore it and this omission rose to a level of deliberate indifference in training their officers. Likewise, in *Johnson v. City of Cincinnati* (1999), policy and training issues stemming from *Monell v. Department* of *Social Services of New York* (1978) were not dismissed. The Court denied summary judgment as the City knew that taking custody of highly agitated people was a recurring problem, and it was aware of the potential risks of placing a person showing sings of delirium in a prone restraint that could result in sudden death.

In *Nelson v. County of Los Angeles* (2003), the decedent's family prevailed in a multi-million dollar judgment when the court agreed that Nelson died from "positional asphyxia." Several deputies responded to a call of a man standing in the street firing a gun at passing motorists. Nelson was controlled, handcuffed with his hands behind his back, and placed in the back seat of the patrol car. He began thrashing in the back seat and the deputies removed him and used the total appendage restraint procedure. Within minutes, Nelson became unresponsive and responding paramedics could not revive him. Despite the fact that Nelson was under the influence of cocaine at the time of arrest and had a history of heart ailments, an expert pathologist opined at trial that these factors did not play a significant part in his death. The pathologist opined that the hogtying position compromised Nelson's ability to breathe and contributed to his death. The court found the county liable for employing the restraint procedure.

In *Price v. County of San Diego* (1998), an arrestee who had a history of methamphetamine use fought violently with police, was restrained in the hogtied position, stopped breathing, and died 2 days later in the hospital. A Section 1983 claim for violation of constitutional rights, wrongful death, and excessive force was filed along with state negligence claims. One medical examiner argued in court that restraint asphyxia contributed to the decedent's death, whereas another medical examiner testified that the hogtied procedure did not dangerously affect oxygen levels, nor did it contribute to the arrestee's death based on medical research concerning restraint asphyxia *(8)*. Based on the medical research, the judge ruled that hogtying, in and of itself, did not cause the arrestee's death and that the deputies did not use excessive force, and acknowledged that the consequences of abusing drugs led to a heart attack, which more than anything killed him. The case was dismissed. In a companion case, *Guseman v. Martinez* (1998), a federal district court in Kansas found that the police officers' method of restraint did not rise to the level of deliberate indifference, despite the arrestee dying in custody, and awarded the City summary judgment.

Similarly. in *Ramirez v. City of Chicago* (1999) and *Tofano v. Reidel* (1999), the courts found in favor of the defendant officers, despite the fact that the arrestees died in restraints. For example, in *Ramirez*, the arrestee had been abusing cocaine and alcohol for 2 days, became paranoid and violent, and fought with a bartender in a bar. Responding officers had to use pepper spray to control him and restrained him with handcuffs. He was placed in the back of the patrol car on his stomach and died during transport to the hospital. In *Tofano,* the subject exhibited extreme agitation and strength, resisted physical efforts of control by several officers, and the application of pepper spray failed. After a struggle with several deputies, they were able to control him and placed him handcuffs. He became unresponsive and died at the hospital. The cause of death was listed as positional asphyxia resulting from the officers' weight on him, toxic levels of cocaine, and congenital heart defect. The court ruled that the deputies acted reasonably.

Likewise, in *Young v. Mt. Rainer* (2001), the court awarded summary judgment to the defendant officers despite Young dying in restraints. Police officers responded to a call that Young was exhibiting bizarre behaviors, was extremely agitated, and upon initial response found him lying on the ground. The officers attempted to take him into custody, but he struggled with them. The officers used pepper spray, and restrained Young with handcuffs and leg restraints. He was transported to the hospital where he died. An autopsy revealed that Young had PCP in his system and the cause of death was listed as sudden cardiac dysrhythmia. Young's parents claimed the officers were deliberately indifferent to his medical needs. The court determined the officers did not violate Young's rights as he struggled and the officers were unaware that he had consumed PCP.

The *Graham* standard of using force is also applied to the reasonable use of restraints in controlling a combative arrestee. Liability attaches only if excessive force that proximately causes injury, in this case death, is used on an individual. The use of restraints must be reasonably related to the behaviors and safety of the individual, the need to control the individual, and the safety concerns of the responding officers. It is standard practice to handcuff arrestee after a force altercation. In combative arrest scenarios (as illustrated by these cases), officers generally need to further restrain the individuals as they frequently will kick and continue their violent behaviors. In response to the citizen's behavior, police officers are authorized to graduate their response to the demands of any particular situation and it is reasonable to handcuff and restrain an individual's legs (*Maynard v. Hopwood*, 1997).

The use of restraints may be considered unreasonable force if they were used inappropriately to the need, officers were not trained in their proper use, or officers failed to follow the department's restraint policy. There must be proof that a particular violation of a federal right was a "highly predictable" consequence of the failure to equip police officers with specific tools to handle recurring situations. The question that emerges from these restraint deaths is whether or not asphyxia deaths are highly foreseeable, predictable, or even occurs as a consequence of restraining persons prone in the hogtie position. The *Graham* standard of objective reasonable force will be applied in restraint cases. The *Price* case is illustrative of this as the court, relying on scientific evidence regarding "hogtying," found the restraint procedure in and of itself not to be excessive force and that it did not cause asphyxia. The court found that drugs caused the individual's death and not the restraint procedure. In analyzing these cases, courts will review the totality of circumstances, cause of death, extent of the person's medical or psychiatric condition, restraints authorized and methods used, other alternatives available, officer's perception of safety, and the resistive behaviors requiring further immobilization of the person. As evidenced in these case examples, the courts are split in their opinions as to whether certain procedures should be considered excessive force and, as litigation is still emerging, changes in court interpretations may be forthcoming.

## Claims of Deliberate Indifference to Medical/Psychological Needs

Beyond the claims of excessive force and improper use of restraints, allegations for failure to recognize behaviors and medical symptoms commonly associated with sudden custodial deaths will be filed. The duty to protect a detainee from harm and to provide reasonable medical care is premised partially on the notion that the government is responsible for these individuals because it has deprived them of the ability to look after themselves (1). The duty begins at arrest and continues through the process of jail custody. The police, however, are not considered absolute ensurers of health to those in their custody. The assertion may be made that officers were deliberately indifferent to the medical/psychological needs of the arrestee. This legal claim may be framed within the context of the Fourteenth Amendment in accordance with the US Supreme Court's decision in *City of Revere v. Massachusetts General Hospital* (1983). This case concluded that municipalities have a constitutional duty to obtain necessary medical care for detainees in their custody. Failing to obtain such care may rise to a level of deliberate indifference.

In *Harris v. District of Columbia* (1991), the estate brought a wrongful death claim under the Fourteenth Amendment alleging that officers were deliberately indifferent to the decedent's medical needs and misused restraints. Harris was "freaking out" on PCP. He was handcuffed, legs restrained, locked in a police van, and was later transported to a hospital. Medical care was delayed at first as a result of filling out forms (per hospital policy), and then it was delayed because the forms were incorrectly completed, according to the attending emergency room physician. Harris was pronounced dead 2 hours and 20 minutes after the arrest in the hospital as a result of a drug overdose. The court held that the police had not entered into a special relationship when they restrained him, and locked him in the van, in that he had not been formally committed, either by conviction, involuntary commitment, or arrest. Thus, there was no duty to obtain medical assistance. Officers were entitled to qualified immunity, as they acted reasonably in light of the circumstances. The court also noted that the officers had not entered into a special relationship requiring a duty to provide medical care, as Harris demonstrated a lack of care for himself when he ingested the PCP. The court's reasoning compared the police officers duty of custody with that of ambulance drivers, stating "they are not subject to a constitutional obligation every time they pick up a patient" (at 15).

In *Cottrell v. Caldwell* (1996), police officers responded to a 911 call and arrested a man with a history of mental illness who stopped taking his medication. The family wanted the officers to transport him to the hospital. After a 20-minute struggle to control the individual, he was subdued, restrained with handcuffs and leg restraints face down on the floor/axle of the car. He was transported to the station and during transport died of "positional asphyxiation." The court, using the deliberate indifference standard, ruled that in "custody mistreatment claims," gross negligence is not part of the standard of review. The standard is deliberate indifference to a "substantial risk of serious harm." The plaintiff must show a deprivation that is "objectively, sufficiently serious," meaning that the officers' actions resulted in the denial of the minimal civilized measure of "life's necessities." The court found no evidence that the officers knew of and consciously disregarded the risk that the arrestee would suffocate, and the plaintiff failed to show a violation of due process. Police did not act with deliberate indifference to the medical and due process rights of the arrestee nor did they use excessive force in restraining him.

In *Simpson v. Hines* (1990), the estate brought a Section 1983 action against 10 officers for alleged excessive force and lack of medical care under the Fourteenth and Fourth Amendments, as well as state claims. The chief of police was sued on grounds of failure to supervise.

After an arrest and confrontation with the deceased, officers were attempting to search him at the station. The arrestee was in a drug-induced state, became violent, and refused to be searched. A struggle ensued, one officer placed him in a "neck hold," while other officers grabbed his arms and legs, and forced him to the floor in order to cuff him. A large officer sat on his chest. After control was established, the arrestee was rolled on his side, handcuffed, with his hands behind his back, and legs restrained. Once restrained, the arrestee became silent, and was left in his cell to recover. During the night, he was checked twice and the officers noted that he did not move from that position. Approximately 5 hours later, an officer noticed a pool of blood near his head and apparently rigor mortis had occurred. The medical examiner reported that the deceased died as a result of asphyxia due to trauma to the neck during struggle to subdue him. On the medical claim, the court held that the officers were deliberately indifferent to the medical needs of the deceased by leaving him unconscious in the cell. The court stated that the officers owe a duty of reasonable care to pretrial detainees under the Fourteenth Amendment.

The applicable standard with regard to medical care issues is deliberate indifference pursuant to *Estelle v. Gamble* (1976). The plaintiff must establish actual omissions sufficiently harmful to evidence deliberate indifference to serious medical needs. To hold officers liable it must be shown that they intentionally denied or delayed access to treatment or interfered with treatment. The Court in *Estelle* held that an inadvertent failure to provide adequate medical care does not rise to a constitutional violation.

The courts do not hold police officers to the same level of care as a medically trained physician, although officers have a responsibility to determine medical or psychological well-being of a person in their custody. The plaintiff may attempt, however, to prove that officers failed to provide medical needs under the ruling in *DeShaney* v. *County of Winnebago* (1989). In this case, the US Supreme Court recognized that a special relationship can exist between the state and a person giving rise to a constitutional duty on the state to assume some responsibility for the person's medical needs only "when the State takes a person into its custody and holds him against his will" ( at 1005). Police officers are under no constitutional obligation to protect or to provide medical services to the general public, even if they know of a particular person's need and regardless of whether state tort law imposes that obligation, unless the government has entered into a "certain special relationships" with the person. When determining whether a "special relationship" may exist for medical purpose, three primary components must be considered, which include the police (a) creating the danger to which plaintiffs were exposed, (b) having knowledge of the impending danger, and (c) having custody of the plaintiff. Hence, liability for police officers may attach when the need for medical care of an arrestee in their custody was created after a force situation (e.g., baton strikes, physical control techniques, during restraint, etc.) and the person sustained an injury, and officers knew that the person needed medical assistance through verbal inquiry or assessment or requests made by the individual. As illustrated in the *Harris* case, medical care liability in sudden in-custody deaths may not attach, as in a significant number of incidents the police take custody and restrain an individual after they have already consumed a quantity of alcohol or recreational drugs. With this in mind, police officers should, however, take reasonable precautions to assess and monitor the condition of the arrestee, and summon medical care as warranted after a violent force restraint confrontation.

## CASE EXAMPLES AGAINST CORRECTION/DETENTION PERSONNEL

### Claims of Excessive Force and Positional Asphyxia

Like their police counterparts, the primary claims filed against the responding officers are allegations of excessive force. In *Bozeman v. Orum* (2002), the estate of the deceased detainee brought a Section 1983 claim against the sheriff and several officers alleging the force used caused his death, thereby violating his Fourteenth Amendment right against the use of excessive force. The detainee had become violent in the jail and the officers had threatened to "kick his ass" if he did not cease. He continued and the officers apparently punched or slapped him. He subsequently died as the result of officers' actions. The court granted summary judgment to the officers and sheriff, noting that some level of force was necessary to restore order where the detainee was going through a mental breakdown in his cell. The court noted that the sheriff had provided adequate training in the proper use of force, including training on positional asphyxia, and was not liable for failing to train or supervise the officers.

Associated with excessive force allegations is a second level of claims that often asserts that the police maximally restrained the deceased, which purportedly contributed to his death. The assertion is frequently made that the deceased died as a result of "positional, postural, restraint, compressional, or mechanical asphyxia," because he was placed in the "hogtied" or restrictive position. The claim may also assert that the individual died from asphyxia as a result of the weight of the officers on his body for an extended period during control and restraint. These allegations may be further supported by results of an autopsy or independent autopsy conducted by a pathologist hired by the estate claiming that the method of restraint contributed to asphyxia, which caused the prisoner's death. Moreover, this assertion will attempt to prove excessive force by utilizing restraints without deference to the obvious medical needs of the prisoner.

One of the first litigated custodial death cases involving the use of restraints in a detention facility is *Lozano v. Smith* (1983). During a pat down, Lozano (who was mentally impaired) struck the arresting officer and violently fought with two officers. One officer struck him in the head with a flashlight, causing a severe injury. Lozano was handcuffed and transported to jail. At booking, he initiated another fight, and several detention officers fought with him and placed him in a padded cell. Later, officers transported him to the emergency room for treatment and medical personnel released him back to the jail. He was placed in a cell and shortly began ramming his head into the cell bars. He was again transported to the hospital, where he stayed for 2 days. He was then released back to the jail and placed in a padded cell. Within a few hours, Lozano began ramming his head into the cell door, causing his head to bleed severely. Lozano had been hitting the door with such force he broke the glass. The sheriff called a doctor and was informed he would be there shortly and would give Lozano a sedative. The sheriff instructed several detention officers to enter the cell to control and restrain Lozano who was screaming and beating his head against the wall. Officers sprayed mace into the cell first but it failed to disable Lozano.

Fearing that Lozano would use a piece of glass to harm himself or them, officers rushed into the cell. One officer placed Lozano in a headlock, while other officers restrained his arms and legs. Lozano grabbed one officer's genitals and began hitting him in the stomach. After a lengthy struggle, officers were able to control and retrain Lozano with handcuffs, hands behind his back. Lozano continued to struggle and a security belt was placed on him. The officers moved Lozano to another cell, but once inside the cell Lozano rammed his head into the wall. Officers took him to the ground and held him down, as he continued to kick and scream. An officer left to obtain leather restraints to secure Lozano's legs. Before the officer returned, an officer with medical experience entered the cell and noticed Lozano's skin turning blue and observed that he was not breathing. The officer initiated CPR and medical personnel responded, but pronounced Lozano dead. An inquest determined that the death was accidental. The autopsy was performed and the pathologist found 115 injuries to Lozano's body, although the pathologist ruled that a significant number were self-precipitated by Lozano. Two doctors stated, however, that Lozano died as a result of traumatic neck injury, which caused asphyxia, and that the fatal neck injury could have been caused by the head-lock placed on Lozano's neck.

Lozano's family filed a Section 1983 claim against the officers for excessive force and claims against the sheriff for failing to train and supervise the officers. Claims of failing to provide medical and psychiatric care were also filed. The court found the sheriff was not liable for Lozano's death nor was liable for a wrongful failure to supervise his officers. The jury found that the officers failed to act in good faith in using the force techniques to subdue Lozano.

*Owens v. City of Atlanta* (1986) is another example of an early custodial restraint death. Owens was arrested for drunk and disorderly and became disruptive in a detention cell at the hospital where he was taken for injuries sustained during his arrest. Officers subdued him and restrained Owens to a bench 12 inches wide running along the back of his cell. His arms were crossed in front of him and cuffed to holes along the bench. His ankles were placed in leg irons and stretched and attached to the holes along the wall. The "stretch-hold position" is called the "mosses crosses." It is a trained restraint technique used only in limited situations with violent detainees. Unable to maintain his balance on the bench, Owens fell forward with his face and shoulders on the floor, and his arms stretched behind him to the bench. When he was discovered, he had a weak pulse and subsequently died. The medical examiner determined he died of positional asphyxia.

The Appellate Court affirmed the lower court's summary judgment decision in favor of the officers. The court noted that the restraint method was not inherently dangerous, the officers had been trained in its use, and had used it before without problem. The officers' action did not rise to a constitutional violation. The court also noted that the agency was not deliberately indifferent to the medical needs of Owens, nor were they indifferent to the training needs regarding the use of the restraints.

## Four-Point Restraint and Pepper Spray

In *Grayson v. Peed* (1999), the Appellate Court affirmed summary judgment for the sheriff and detention officers in restraint death incident where physical force and pepper spray were used and the detainee was placed in a four-point restraint position (supine with ankles and wrists restrained to a bed). The estate of the deceased detainee charged under Section 1983 that the sheriff had failed to supervise and train the officers in the proper use of force and equipment, thereby violating the constitutional rights of the prisoner. During booking, the intoxicated detainee acted irrationally, and began yelling and screaming. He was stripped searched, placed in a cell, and a struggle ensued. Officers used pepper spray to control him and he calmed down. The next morning he became violent again and an extraction team of five officers forcibly removed him to another cell after he refused to cooperate. He was sprayed and punched several times by officers during the cell extraction. He was restrained, re-located, and placed in a four-point restraint position. He was monitored and within minutes he appeared to be unconscious, but felt to be "fine" by medical personnel. Shortly thereafter, an officer noticed he was not breathing, CPR was initiated, and he was transported to the local hospital where he expired. He died of congestive heart failure due to an enlarged heart.

The Appellate Court granted summary judgment to the sheriff and officers ruling that their use of force was necessitated by the detainee's behaviors and was used in good faith to control the detainee. The court also noted that the sheriff was not deliberately indifferent to the medical needs of the detainee. The Court stated there was a trained medic on hand during booking and during the encounter, and he responded appropriately once the need for medical care became apparent. Furthermore, the court noted that the detention facility had been accredited by the American Corrections Association and the National Commission on Correctional Health Care for 10 years and no actionable deficiencies in the policies, customs, or training were evident.

The jury returned a "no cause" for action verdict in *Love v. Bolinger* (1998). During a hearing to determine the competency to stand trial of a bipolar individual, the detainee became agitated and rushed the judge's bench. Five officers struggled with the detainee and sprayed him twice with pepper spray. Once he was finally subdued, two sets of handcuffs were secured with his hands in front. He was escorted from the courtroom, down one floor, to a padded cell in the detention center. The detainee continued to struggle during the escort and fought with officers, kicking them once they placed him in the cell. While officers were removing the handcuffs, one officer noticed he had stopped breathing, and began CPR, while another officer summoned medical personnel. Within several minutes, paramedics responded and continued lifesaving efforts. A pulse was restored but it stopped during transport to the hospital, where he was pronounced dead. The estate filed a Section 1983 action claiming he died of asphyxiation from a chokehold and the officers placing their weight on him in the cell. Two other pathologists reviewed the autopsy and each determined he died of an enlarged heart. Over 5 days, the jury listened to the officers' and expert witness testimony. They found in favor of the officers, finding they did not use excessive force, nor did they cause the death of the decedent.

## Deliberate Indifference to Obvious Medical/Psychological Needs

The duty to protect a detainee from harm and to provide reasonable medical care is premised partially on the notion that the government is responsible for these individuals because it has deprived them of the ability to care for themselves *(1)*. The applicable standard with regard to medical care issues is "deliberate indifference" pursuant to *Estelle v. Gamble* (1976) in accordance with the Eighth Amendment. The plaintiff must establish actual omissions sufficiently harmful to evidence deliberate indifference to serious medical needs. In *Estelle,* the Court held that an inadvertent failure to provide adequate medical care does not rise to a constitutional violation. Corrections officers, however, are not considered absolute ensurers of health to those in their custody. The courts do not hold detention/corrections officers to the same level of care as a medically trained physician, although officers have a responsibility to determine medical or psychological well-being of a person in their custody.

In many of these violent restraint situations, the prisoner is mentally impaired, has had a history of prescribed antipsychotic medication use (but may have not taken it recently), or is currently abusing recreational drugs. In many of these incidents, the prisoner's overall health condition is extremely poor, as the prisoner may have a diseased heart and defects of other internal organs. Officers also encounter those individuals who are under the influence of a chemical at time of booking and become violent or shortly after a period of incarceration, require restraint, and suddenly die. With this in mind, officers should take reasonable precautions to assess and monitor the condition of the prisoner and summon medical care as warranted after a violent force restraint confrontation.

Prisoners who have consumed a quantity of drugs prior to police contact may have been confined in jail. These individuals may have consumed the drugs so that they would not get caught with an illegal substance in their possession. Within hours after confinement, they may develop a drug-induced condition known as excited/agitated delirium *(9)*. Depending on the dose and the chronicity of use, observable behaviors can include hallucinations, incoherent speech, violent behaviors, a high threshold to pain, increased strength, and constant purposeless activity *(10)*. Excited delirium is usually considered a medical emergency, but with a psychiatric presentation *(11)*. Corrections officers encounter prisoners who may be tearing up their cells, or have become violent, and self-injurious, requiring officers to physically control them.

In *Hoyer v. City of Southfield and County of Oakland* (2003), five officers were dispatched to contain a mentally impaired, partially clothed man who was running at cars in the. He violently fought with the officers, requiring one officer to use three baton strikes, another to spray two bursts of pepper spray, and another officer to use a brachial stun to the neck, and several knee strikes to Hoyer's thigh, in order to subdue him. Three of the officers sustained injuries and were treated at the hospital. Hoyer was transported to the jail, where, within 20 minutes of being placed in a cell, he began banging his head on the wall, shouting, and attempting to pull the toilet from the wall. Paramedics were called and an extraction team removed Hoyer from his cell. Once in the ambulance, he became unresponsive and later died at the hospital. The estate filed a legal action, claiming, excessive force and deliberate indifference to Hoyer's medical condition. The autopsy revealed that Hoyer died as a result of acute cocaine intoxication (4 g in his system) and agitated delirium. The Court granted summary judgment to both defendants. Neither defendant was deliberately indifferent to Hoyer's medical condition nor used excessive force in subduing him.

In *Smith v. Wilson County* (2000), Smith died of cocaine intoxication in the detention center and his family filed a Section 1983 action for failing to provide medical care at time of arrest and while confined. Smith resisted arrest for failing to stop at a stop sign. Officers noticed he was chewing something and he attempted to remove it. Smith stated he swallowed a marijuana cigarette, and then said it was rock cocaine, and then said it was marijuana. The arresting officer asked if he wanted medical attention, Smith refused, and he was transported to the police department for processing. At the station, Smith informed the lieutenant that he had not swallowed cocaine. The lieutenant instructed the officer to take Smith to the magistrate. The magistrate set Smith's bond and Smith did not complain about needing medical care nor did he appear to be under the influence of drugs. He was booked into the detention center, being unable to post bond. Smith was placed in a holding cell and shortly became agitated and began yelling. Officers moved him to an isolation cell and Smith stated that the "rock of cocaine he swallowed is killing me." Smith then stated he only swallowed a marijuana cigarette. Officers did not summon medical personnel, as Smith did not appear to need medical treatment.

During a standard security check 3 hours later, Smith was found unconscious in his cell. Medical personnel were summoned and life-saving efforts was initiated but unsuccessful and Smith was pronounced dead at the hospital, approximately 5 hours after he was arrested. The autopsy revealed that Smith had not suffered any "acute external injuries." The pathologist determined the cause of death to be from cocaine intoxication, which caused an idiosyncratic reaction of the heart because Smith's heart was enlarged from extensive cocaine abuse.

The family filed a legal action claiming the arresting officers used excessive force in taking Smith to the ground and were deliberately indifferent in failing to provide medical care in violation of his Fourth and Fourteenth Amendments. The court awarded summary judgment to the arresting officers. The family also filed claims against the detention facility officers and the sheriff, for wrongful death, officers failing to recognize and respond to a medical emergency, and failing to train, supervise, and direct officers in the care of intoxicated prisoners, under the Fourteenth Amendment. The Court granted summary judgment to the detention personnel also, finding no evidence that the officers or the sheriff were deliberately indifferent to Smith's medical needs.

## CASE EXAMPLES OF FAILURE TO TRAIN RESPONDING PERSONNEL

A frequent claim in unexpected death actions are allegations that supervisors failed to train officers. The assertion is that officers have not been instructed or trained properly by the supervisor or agency and thus lack the skills, knowledge, or competency required in a range of items, such as use of appropriate force measures including the use of restraints and other equipment, recognizing the hazards of drug-induced violent behavior, deficiency in training to obvious medical or psychiatric behaviors, recognizing the risks of restraints, and a lack of training in policies and procedures for responding to special needs prisoners (those intoxicated or mentally impaired).

Section 1983 claims of this nature will focus on the US Supreme Court case of *City of Canton v. Harris* (1989). The Court established the inadequacy of police training may serve as a basis for Section 1983 liability only where the failure to train amounts to deliberate indifference to the rights of persons with whom the police come into contact. The plaintiff must show that the custom or policy of the department was to ignore officer training and this was the moving force behind a constitutional violation. In custodial death cases, the plaintiff must show that the alleged lack of training with regard to the use of force and restraints and the alleged lack of medical/psychiatric care for special needs prisoners, is closely related and actually caused the officers deliberate indifference to the serious medical needs of the arrestee.

### Failure-to-Train Claims Against the Police

In *Elmes v. Hart* (1994), an estate filed a Section 1983 and state tort claims when an arrestee high on LSD and marijuana died in police custody. Officers responded to a disturbance at a party where they observed the deceased choking a female guest. After an intense struggle, several officers were needed to subdue the violent male. Handcuffs and leg restraints were secured on the kicking arrestee, and he was hogtied with flex cuffs and leg restraints. The medical examiner was summoned to the scene and found the arrestee hogtied and learned he had stopped breathing after several minutes of being hogtied. An ambulance was summoned, but there was no attempt at resuscitation, as there was no CPR mask available, and officers were fearful of contracting a transmissible disease such as AIDS. They had felt for a pulse and finding none thought CPR would be futile. The autopsy report cited death was caused by "mechanical asphyxiation." The court ruled that the officers did not "intentionally kill the arrestee." An excessive force claim was made against the officers in which the Court found that the officers did use excessive force in arresting the deceased. The City, however, was not found to be deliberately indifferent for failing to train its officers.

In *Pilakos v. City of Manchester, New Hampshire* (2003), the court held that physically controlling a combative subject who twice kicked and beat off a police dog, fought with several officers, fought through a 2-second burst of pepper spray, was not unreasonable nor excessive force. After Pilakos was restrained, he remained on his stomach for approximately 3 minutes, became unresponsive, and later died. Pilakos suffered from bipolar affective disorder, an enlarged heart, and was under the influence of cocaine during the confrontation. Pilakos' estate claimed that the chief failed to train officers in properly restraining agitated persons and monitoring them while in restraints. The court reasoned that, in light of the circumstances, the officers did not violate their training and it was not unreasonable to keep Pilakos on his stomach restrained for his and the officers safety.

Conversely, in *Cruz v. City of Laramie, Wyoming* (2001), the Tenth Circuit Court found that hogtying individuals with diminished capacity was excessive force and denied summary judgment for the City of Laramie. Cruz was found by officers to be naked and running wildly. Believing he was on some type of drug, officers summoned an ambulance and verbal calming attempts were unsuccessful. He fought with the officers and they restrained him with handcuffs, and because he was kicking, a nylon strap was placed on his ankles and connected to the handcuffs. Cruz calmed down, but officers noticed his face had blanched and removed the restraints. Emergency medical personnel initiated CPR and Cruz died at the hospital. An autopsy revealed a large amount of cocaine in his system. His family filed a civil action claiming he died of restraint asphyxia, which was supported by one medical expert, whereas another medical expert claimed his death was solely from cocaine abuse.

A dispute emerged over whether Cruz was hogtied or hobbled. The lower court determined that had the officers separated Cruz's ankles further from his restrained hands, by 2 feet or more, Cruz would have been hobbled. The Court reasoned that the hogtied restraint technique does not *per se* constitute a constitutional right violation, rather officers may not apply the technique when an individual's diminished capacity is apparent. Such diminished capacity may result from intoxication, the influence of controlled substances, a discernable mental condition, or any other condition apparent to officers. The Appellate Court ruled that the officers knew Cruz was under the influence and using the hogtie restraint amounted to excessive force. Liability attached against the City for failing to train officers in the use of hobble restraints.

## Failure-to-Train Claims Against Correction/Detention Officers

In *Swans v. City of Lansing* (1998), the jury found in favor of the plaintiff who died in a detention cell. Upon being admitted into the detention center, Swans kicked the booking sergeant in the head and fought with officers. He was restrained with handcuffs, but the officers were unable to secure him in a restraint chair. He was forcibly moved to a cell where he continued to violently fight with the officers. In the cell, five officers and a lieutenant attempted to further restrain him with a kick-stop restraint strap, like they had used in numerous other situations with violent detainees. The strap broke and the officers restrained Swans with additional handcuffs and leg-irons connected to his ankles. The officers left Swans on his side/stomach, monitored him by closed-circuit television, and returned to the cell within 10 minutes. The officers found Swans lying in urine and unresponsive. They moved him to the hallway, removed the restraints, initiated CPR, and summoned medical personnel. Medical personnel found him pulseless, continued life-saving efforts, and transported him to the hospital, where he was pronounced dead. An autopsy revealed that he died from cardiac dysrhythmia caused by postural asphyxia, during custodial restraint. The jury determined that officers used excessive force, misused the restraints, and that administrative personnel had failed to train, supervise, and direct officers in how to properly respond and restraint mentally impaired detainees. The jury awarded $10 million to Swans' estate.

The use of restraints may be considered unreasonable force if they are used inappropriately to the need, officers were not trained in their proper use, or officers failed to follow the department's restraint policy. There must be proof that a particular violation of a federal right was a "highly predictable" consequence of the failure to equip police officers with specific tools to handle recurring situations. The question that emerges from these restraint deaths is whether or not asphyxia deaths are highly foreseeable, predictable, or even occur as a consequence of restraining persons prone. The question of whether supervisors were deliberately indifferent to the training of their officers in the use of restraints with special needs prisoners also emerges.

In *Sims v. Greenville, County* (2000), a detainee was being moved from a holding area to a holding cell in order to serve a meal. The detainee resisted the detention officers, and four officers took him the floor. One officer applied a chokehold on the fighting detainee. The detainee was maximally restrained with handcuffs and leg restraints and placed in the holding cell. The detainee became unresponsive and attempts of medical intervention were unsuccessful. He later died and the pathologist determined that the cause of death was positional asphyxia. The detainee's family filed a legal action claiming that the officers used excessive force and inappropriately used a "multiple officer take-down" technique. Claims against the sheriff alleged that he failed to train officers and instituted an unconstitutional policy of using a multi-officer take-down maneuver. The Appellate Court affirmed summary judgment by the lower court, determining that the estate failed to present evidence that the defendants used excessive force. The estate failed to show that the sheriff maintained unconstitutional policies that would subject detainees to excessive force measures.

As previously discussed, in *Grayson v. Peed* (1999), *Bozeman v. Orum* (2002), *Love v. Bolinger* (1998), *Hoyer v. Southfield and County of Oakland* (2003), and *Sims v. Greenville County* (2002), the courts determined that claims of failure to train failed to rise to a level of deliberate indifference. In *Grayson*, the court noted that the detention facility had been accredited by the American Corrections Association and the National Commission on Correctional Health Care for 10 years and no actionable deficiencies in the policies, customs, or training were evident. Furthermore, in *Bozeman*, the court noted that the sheriff had developed a policy on use of force and recognizing special needs detainees, provided adequate training in the proper use of force, including training on positional asphyxia, and was not liable for failing to train or supervise the officers. Likewise, in *Sims*, the court ruled that the officers had been trained in the proper multi-officer take-down technique, trained in the use-of-force policy, trained to avoid placing a knee on a detainee's neck, and trained in factors relative to positional asphyxia. Hence, allegations that the sheriff failed to train his officers did not survive. Moreover, failure to train claims did not prevail in the *Love* and *Hoyer* cases, as administrators had provided adequate training in the use of force, restraints, other force equipment, and responding to the mentally impaired.

With increased frequency, correctional agencies are using a restraint chair to further restrain a violent prisoner. It can provide a humane method for restraining the combative prisoner, which allows the prisoner time to calm down for self-protection and the protection for officers, other prisoners, and attending medical personnel *(12)*. Claims of excessive force and failing to train officers in the proper use of the chair have been filed as a result of the deaths of several prisoners. In *Jones v. Devaney* (2004) and *Bishop v. Corsentino* (2004), prisoners became combative requiring officers to further restrain them in the restraint chair because of their continued self-injurious behaviors. The prisoners were placed in the chair, monitored, and later became unresponsive. Lifesaving efforts were initiated and both prisoners died as a result of unspecified medical conditions. In both cases, the courts granted summary judgment as it was shown that the officers were guided in the proper use of the chair by agency policy. Training in the policy and the mechanics of using the chair was provided by the agency and the policy also provided for officer monitoring and intervals of medical personnel assessment. In both cases, the procedures and officer training was followed, and the courts determined that the use of the chair failed to amount to excessive force in restraining the violent prisoners.

The use of restraints may be considered unreasonable force if they are used inappropriately to the need, if officers are not trained in their proper use, or if officers fail to follow the department's restraint policy. There must be proof that a particular violation of a federal right was a "highly predictable" consequence of the failure to equip police officers with specific tools to handle recurring situations. The question emerges of whether supervisors were deliberately indifferent to the training of their officers in the use of restraints with special needs prisoners.

The *Price* case is illustrative of this as the court, relying on scientific evidence regarding "hogtying," found the restraint procedure in and of itself not to be excessive force and that it did not cause asphyxia. The court found that drugs caused the individual's death and not the restraint procedure. The *Swans* case, however, reveals how a jury may view this phenomenon, despite the reliable scientific research showing that maximally restraining a violent mentally impaired person is not in and of itself deadly force. In analyzing these cases, courts will review the totality of circumstances, cause of death, extent of the person's medical or psychiatric condition, restraints authorized and methods used, officer's perception of safety, and the resistive behaviors requiring further immobilization of the person. As evidenced in these case examples, the courts are more likely to grant summary judgment to the officers and/or correctional agencies, when they can justify the appropriate level of force, based on the circumstances facing them, and when the officers have been provided with proper training, and guided by sound policy.

## CONCLUDING OBSERVATIONS

Wrongful death allegations in sudden in-custody deaths are an emerging topic area of liability in policing and corrections. Although rare, the liability potential for a wrongful death from sudden in-custody deaths can be significant. Law enforcement officers and administrators possess a broad range of responsibilities with detainees in their custody. The police and correction officers are not absolute guarantors of health, but they do owe a degree of care for those arrestees in their custody who otherwise cannot care for themselves under theories of negligence and Section 1983 provisions.

Based on case analysis, criminal justice agencies can insulate their officers and themselves from liability by taking a proactive stance in considering the following policy and training recommendations. As these arrest situations allege excessive force, administrators are encouraged to first review and revise their use of force policy to insure that officers are directed in using "objective reasonable" force in accordance with court holdings. It should direct officers in the proper escalation and de-escalation in a variety of physical force techniques and equipment based on the behaviors manifested by the arrestee. Included in the force policy should be a section devoted to the use of authorized restraints. This section should direct officers in utilizing department issued restraint devices that specify how to further restrain combative and special needs detainees.

Procedures that direct officers in responding to the mentally or chemically impaired (special needs detainees) need to be revised or developed . This policy should be structured within state standards for dealing with detainees who require medical or psychiatric treatment or hospitalization and how transportation will occur. The policy should direct officers in how to respond to this population, when to summon back-up or a supervisor, when to summon medical or psychological assistance, and to what facility these individuals should be transported. Proper response and precautions employed with at-risk detainees commences with policies that direct officers in justifiable decisions when encountering such individuals. These issues need to be examined and addressed pursuant to policy prior to the need arising.

## REFERENCES

1. Silver I. Police Civil Liability. Matthew Bender, Newark, NJ, 2001.
2. Ross DL. Civil Liability in Criminal Justice. Anderson Publishing, Cincinnati, OH, 2003.
3. del Carmen RV. Civil Liabilities in American Policing: A Text for Law Enforcement Personnel. Brady, Englewood Cliffs, NJ, 1991.
4. Kappeler V. Critical Issues in Police Civil Liability (3rd ed.). Waveland Press, Prospect Heights, IL, 2001.
5. Ross DL. Assessing in-custody deaths in Jails. American Jails 2001;25(4):13–26.
6. Kappeler V, Vaughn M, del Carmen RV. Death in detention: An analysis of police liability for negligent failure to prevent suicide. J Crim Justice 1991;19:381–393.

7. del Carmen RV, Kappeler V. Municipal and police agencies as defendants: liability for official policy and custom. Am J Police 1991;10:1–17.

8. Chan T, Vilke G, Neuman T, Clausen J. Restraint position asphyxia. Ann Emerg Med 1997;30:578–586.

9. Ruttenber AJ, Lawler-Heavner J, Ming Y, Wetli CV, Hearn WL, Mash DC. Fatal excited delirium following cocaine use: epidemiologic findings provide new evidence for mechanics of cocaine toxicity. J Forensic Sci 1997;42:25–31.

10. Ross DL. Factors associated with excited delirium deaths in police custody. Mod Pathol 1998;11:1127–1137.

11. Wetli CV, Fishbain DA. Cocaine-induced psychosis and sudden death in recreational Cocaine users. J Forensic Sci 1985;30:873–880.

12. DeLand GW. Restraint chairs, part I: reasonable control aid or the devil's chair? Corrections Managers' Report 2000;3:33–43.

## CASES CITED

*Abrhams v. Mayes*, 436 So. 2d 1099 (LA Dist. Crt. App. 1983)

*Animashaun v. O'Donnell*, No 91C2632 (N.D. Ill., 1994)

*Bell v. Wolfish*, 441 U.S. 520 (1979)

*Bishop v. Corsentino*, 371 F.3d 1203 (10th Cir. 2004)

*Bozeman v. Orum*, 199 F. Supp. 2d 1216 (M.D. Ala. 2002)

*Brinkman v. City of Indianapolis*, 231, N.E. 2d 169 (Ind. Ct. App. 1967)

*Brown v. Lee*, 639, So.2d 897 (LA App.1994)

*City of Canton v. Harris*, 489 U.S. 378 (1989)

*City of Revere v. Massachusetts General Hospital*, 463 U.S. 239 (1983)

*Cottrell, v. Caldwell*, 85 F. 3rd 1480 (11th Cir. 1996)

*Cruz v. City of Laramie, WY*, 239 F.3d 1183 (10th Cir. 2001)

*Del Tufo v. Township of Old Bridge*, 685 A.2d 1267 (N.J. 1996)

*DeShaney v. Winnebago County Department of Social Services*, 489 U.S. 189 (1989)

*East v. City of Chicago*, 719 F. Supp. 683 (N.D. Ill. 1989)

*Elmes v. Hart*, 03A01-9319-CV-00372 (Tenn. Ct. App., 1994)

*Estelle v. Gamble*, 429 U.S. 97 (1976)

*Estate of Phillips v. City of Milwaukee*, 928 F. Supp. 817 (E.D. Wis. 1996)

*Farmer v. Brennan*, 511 U.S. 285 (1994)

*Fruge v. City of New Orleans*, 613 So. 2nd 811 (LA Dist. Ct. App. 1993)

*Graham v. Connor*, U.S. 190 S. Ct. 1865 (1989)

*Guseman v. Martinez*, 1998 WL 166235 (D. Kan. 1998))

*Grayson v. Peed*, 195 F. 3d 692 (4th Cir. 1999)

*Gregoire v. Class*, 236 F. 3d 413 (8th Cir. 2000)

*Harris v. District of Columbia*, 932 F.2d 10 (D.C. Cir. 1991)

*Hoyer v. City of Southfield and County of Oakland*, No. 01-CV-70643-DT (E.D. S. Mi., 2003) [unpublished]

*Hudson v. McMillian*, 503 U.S. 1 (1992)

*Johnson v. City of Cincinnati*, 39 F. Supp. 2d 1013, 1018-1020 (S.D. Ohio 1999)

*Johnson v. Glick,* 481 F. 2d 1028 (2nd Cir.1973)

*Jones v. Devaney*, No. 03-15744, Lexis 13700 (9th Cir. 2004) [unpublished]
*Lozano v. Smith*, 718 F. 2d 756 (5th Cir. 1983)
*Love v. Bolinger*, IP 95-1465-C-B/S, Ind. (1998) [unpublished]
*Maynard v. Hopwood,* 105 F. 3d 1226 (8th Cir. 1997)
*Monell v. Department of Social Services of NY*, 436 U.S. 658 (1978)
*Nelson v. Los Angles County*, 2d App. Dist. Div. 1, No. B161431103
*Owens v. City of Atlanta*, 780 F. 2d 1564 (11th Cir. 1986)
*Pilakos v. City of Manchester, New Hampshire*, No. 01-461-M (DNH (2003)
*Price v. County of San Diego*, 990 F. Supp. 1230 (S.D. Cal.1998)
*Ramirez v. City of Chicago,* 82 F. F. Supp. 2d 836 (N.D. Ill. 1999)
*Rochin v. California*, 342 U.S. 165 (1952)
*Shuff v. Zurich*, 173 So. 2d 393 (LA Ct. App. 1965)
*Simpson v. Hines*, 903 F. 2d 400 (5th Cir. 1990)
*Sims v. Greenville County,* 221 F. 3d 1265 (4th Cir. 2000)
*Smith v. Wilson County*, No. 5:98-CV-842-BO (3) (E.D. N.C., 2000) [unpublished]
*Swans v. City of Lansing*, 65 F. Supp. 2d 625 (W. D. Mich. 1998)
*Tennessee v. Garner* 471 U.S. 1 (1985)
*Thomas v. Williams*, 124 S.E.2d 409 (GA App. 1962)
*Tindall v. Multnomah County*, 570 P.2d 979 (OR App. 1977)
*Toano v. Reidel,* 61 F. Supp. 2d 289 (D.N.J.1999)
*Wagar v. Hasenkrug*, 486, F. Supp. 47 (D. Mont.1980)
*Wright v. Collins*, 766 F.2d 841 (5th Cir. 1985)
*Young v. City of Mount Rainer*, 238 F. 3d 567 (4th Cir. 2001)

# Chapter 12

# Administrative Implications

## Darrell L. Ross

The diverse nature and importance of this subject matter create a number of administrative implications for law enforcement managers, trainers, and line officers. The preceding chapters have described the complexity of sudden in-custody deaths by explaining the nature of the problem, the physiological, psychological, and pharmacological issues, use-of-force and restraint concerns, liability issues, and investigation issues. Collectively, administrative personnel in police and correctional agencies, who can direct their line officers in how to best respond to these encounters, should address these factors. In order to place their agencies in the best position to defend against a litigation claim associated with a sudden in-custody death, administrators should also address these issues.

The purpose of this chapter is to describe a proactive systematic approach to managing a law enforcement agency's response to violent physical use-of-force encounters. Because of the complexity of the subject and the numerous factors involved in these encounters, officers clearly need direction to ensure they are following their agency's use-of-force training and policies, case law decisions, and are making justifiable decisions in determining the appropriate course of action in varying situations. Deliberating how to best respond during the course of a violent restraint situation is not the appropriate time to discover that officers are not prepared to handle the situation as a result of training or policy deficiencies, or a lack of the appropriate equipment with which to respond to the situation. Hence, by assessing the subject matter and topics of the previous chapters of this text, administrators are encouraged to develop and implement the recommended strategies presentedbased on the needs facing an individual agency.

From: *Forensic Science and Medicine: Sudden Deaths in Custody*
Edited by: D. L. Ross and T. C. Chan © Humana Press Inc., Totowa, NJ

## ADOPTING A RISK MANAGEMENT APPROACH

Generally, incidents of sudden in-custody deaths revolve around four broad areas:

1. The degree and type of force/restraint measures officers used to control and restrain the violent subject.
2. The medical and/or psychological factors associated with the death of the subject.
3. The medical care issues provided or requested by responding officers.
4. The method used for transporting the subject.

Because sudden in-custody deaths center on the reasonableness of the use-of-force techniques and equipment officers decide to use for restraint, developing a comprehensive use-of-force management system is suggested.

As mentioned throughout this text, sudden in-custody deaths after restraint are rare in occurrence in police and correctional contexts. Although the frequency of such an event is rare, the severity of such an occurrence is high, normally resulting in an extensive investigation and a multi-million dollar lawsuit *(1)*. An important place to start to apply the information identified in this text is to adopt a risk management perspective in creating a use-of-force management system. The ongoing process of risk management involves assessing prior encounters to plan how to reduce and control future occurrences. Risk management builds on fundamental managerial functions such as planning, organizing, controlling, budgeting, staffing, allocating resources, reporting, and evaluation. Risk management adds to these managerial dimensions through an ongoing process of incident analysis, job assessments, identifying risk exposure, forecasting, controlling resources, loss reduction, loss prevention/avoidance, selecting appropriate risk-reduction strategies, policy development/implementation, training, operational monitoring, and assessment. Risk management can assist in controlling risks, managing costs of the agency, reducing loss, and defending lawsuits *(2)*.

Risk management is not just an administrative function, but fundamentally involves all personnel within an agency that promotes a proactive approach to efficient organizational operations. The components of risk management provide several layers of protection that can increase officer safety and provides a framework whereby officers and administrators work together to implement risk-control strategies. Risk management cannot eliminate all risks of the job or lawsuits, but assists members of law enforcement and detention agencies in forming a system with which to address common and potential circumstances that pose a critical problem.

### *Stage 1: Incident Analysis*

Establishing a risk management program that addresses violent use-of-force restraint situations involves several stages. Analyzing past incidents and case decisions of sudden in-custody deaths comprise the first stage. Chapters 3–6, 8, and 9 provided an assessment and description of the medical, physiological, and substance abuse factors associated with these deaths. Chapter 11 also described liability issues associated with incidents of in-custody deaths. These chapters provide an excellent foundation with which to assess subjects who may manifest symptoms consistent with in-custody restraint deaths. The information contained within these chapters can assist in developing policy, providing training, and properly performing field operations when officers encounter such an arrest or control circumstance.

Moreover, administrators are encouraged to analyze their own agency arrest incident records, use-of-force reports, and local community hospital emergency room records in order to determine the frequency of contact with subjects who are under the influence of varying substances or who exhibit mental impairment. In some communities, this population comprises a significant number of police contacts, calls for service, and emergency room services. For example, in 2003, Bell and Kissin *(3)* reported that from 1994 to 2001, about 5% of all hospital emergency room admissions were for subjects who were abusing drugs. Seven categories accounted for 85% of the admissions in 2001: alcohol (34%), cocaine (30%), marijuana (17%), benzodiazephines (16%), narcotic analegics/combainations (28%), heroin (15%), and antidepressants (10%). Police have a higher probability of contacting these individuals than others in the community. Moreover, in many jurisdictions, police officers frequently have contact with mentally impaired persons who manifest violent tendencies toward themselves, others, or the responding officers. The nature and frequency of police contact with this population should also be assessed.

Furthermore, detention facility personnel are encouraged to analyze their own admission records and/or incident reports in order to identify the frequency of confining the mentally impaired and subjects under the influence of a chemical. Previous studies performed on the prevalence of severe mental illness among incarcerated populations estimate a range from 8 to 16% *(4–6)*. Beck and Maruschak *(7)* reported that more than 16% of jail detainees were identified as mentally impaired, 30% exhibited a history of alcohol dependence, 60% were under the influence of alcohol or other substance at the time of committing the offense, and 50% took medication during their confinement.

Analyzing 3 to 5 years worth of calls for service, incidents, or admissions where officers responded to these two types of populations can assist in determining the frequency and severity (criticality) of the contacts between officers and these subjects. The frequency and severity index should be used when performing an incident analysis. Frequency refers to the actual number of occurrences of an incident. Severity refers to the criticality of the outcome of the incident by assessing the potential for loss, dollar loss, injury, death, damage result, and the potential for incurring a lawsuit. Typically, the association between frequency and severity results in an inverse relationship. For example, although the number of police contacts, calls for service, or jail admissions of these two types of populations may be frequent, a sudden in-custody death after a restraint encounter is highly rare, but can be observed as critical or severe. The severity focuses on questions of the reasonableness of the force measures officers used, what caused or contributed to the death, and whether the restraining officers and/or their supervisors should be held responsible for the person's death.

Another important component in this stage is to consider the principle of foreseeability, which brings the components of frequency and severity into sharper focus. When assessing frequency and severity of an incident, two questions can be asked: "What is the foreseeability or the likelihood of the officer contacting or confining a subject in this population?" "How does the nature of the contact relate to frequency and severity?" Depending on the findings of the analysis, foreseeability may underscore frequency and severity, suggesting that such encounters should be addressed through risk management strategies. In many communities, the frequency of contact with individuals under the influence of a chemical substance and/or who are mentally impaired is moderate to high, necessitating the need to address the issue through risk management strategies.

## Stage 2: Policy Development

Once an incident analysis has been performed, the next stage is to develop or revise departmental policy that will address the issue of responding to these two types of populations. As the majority of contacts with these subjects may revolve around issues of use of force, it is suggested that the department's use-of-force policy be expanded or revised to address not only the appropriate force measures officers should employ but also to include other components (i.e., monitoring/medical care issues, methods for transport, etc.) that are usually associated with a sudden in-custody restraint death.

The role of policy indicates to the public where an agency stands on major issues, while concomitantly providing department personnel with guidance and direction in decision making. A policy is a means by which an agency can guide the actions, authority, and decisions of its officers. The goal of developing policy is not to totally eliminate an officer's discretion, but rather to establish a framework in which to make decisions. Policies should be based on and reflect statutes, state standards, and court decisions as they operationalize legislation and court holdings into agency practices. Policies provide guides to an officer's thinking, whereas procedures guide an officer's actions. Procedures should be developed that (a) describe the methods for performing a task or operation and (b) identifies the personnel responsible for carrying out the action. Procedures should be written in a manner that provides flexibility of officer response or actions.

From a risk management perspective, policies and procedures provide the first line of defense against potential litigation. Revising and developing policies and procedures is an administrative function and complies with the US Supreme Court's decision in *Monell v. New York Department of Social Services* (1978). Administrators can incur liability for failing to direct officers, which can be interpreted as a lack of direction and guidance through written policies and procedures. A broadly written use-of-force policy not only assists in officer decision making and authorizing measures and equipment to employ, but it can also assist in the reduction of allegations of excessive force, brutality, and wrongful in-custody deaths. The policy can also serve as a training tool and can most assuredly assist in defending a claim of a wrongful sudden in-custody death where allegations of excessive force have been filed. A policy or procedure should be attentive to the four Cs: current, comprehensive, consistent, and constitutional. Components of a use-of-force policy are described later in this chapter.

## Stage 3: Risk Control

The next stage involves selecting a risk-control strategy or combinations of strategies to control the risk. Possible risk-control strategies include risk avoidance, risk transfer, loss prevention, loss reduction, segregation of resources, and training. Risk avoidance involves an agency voluntarily deciding not to undertake a certain activity. For example, a police department may decide not to provide motorcade escort services in a funeral procession owing to lack of personnel or safety issues. Because policing and confining detainees requires certain job requirements, complete risk avoidance is not always an option for criminal justice personnel or agencies. Detention centers, however, frequently require medical clearance from a physician prior to admitting a detainee exhibiting an obvious injury. Instituting such a policy has averted risk for detention personnel.

Risk transfer is related to risk avoidance, but involves making a decision to move or transfer the risk of a task from one party to another. In policing, this may include an officer transporting a mentally impaired arrestee to a hospital for psychiatric evaluation and clearance prior to transporting the individual to jail. It may include summoning emergency medical personnel to an arrest scene or a jail cell to provide emergency medical care to an injured arrestee or detainee. Another example may be to summon medical personnel to transport a violent or injured arrestee to the hospital instead of in a patrol vehicle. This strategy controls risks by identifying situations (based on the outcome of stage 1) in which an agency or an officer can transfer risk to another party prior to incurring a loss.

The strategy of loss prevention institutes measures prior to an incident occurring. The goal is to prevent the frequency of the loss-causing event. Generally, this can mean establishing and implementing departmental policies and procedures, conducting in-service training, authorizing issuing appropriate equipment, maintaining equipment and vehicles by keeping them functional, and equipping vehicles with protective screens and hazard-free back seats. In detention centers, this may include maintaining functional observation cells, closed-circuit cameras in cells, and security checks (training is discussed in a separate section of this chapter).

Loss reduction differs from loss prevention by attempting to minimize a loss, rather than preventing it. Examples of loss reduction in policing include requiring multiple officers to respond to certain types of calls or to serve commitment papers and providing officers with various less lethal force options. In detention centers instituting admission practices, screening detainees regarding medical and psychological needs, and maintaining access to health care personnel may not totally prevent a detainee from injuring him or herself or dying, but may assist in reducing the frequency of occurrence.

Segregating resources provides for maintaining agency resources in varying locations so that no single incident depreciates the use of the equipment. The objective is to reduce the severity of potential losses allowing the officer or agency the ability to function. It can include maintaining back-up equipment such as restraint devices, other force equipment, back-up vehicles, spare equipment, facilities, overlapping shifts, cross-training of officers, and using overflow cells, where feasible. It may consist of authorizing only patrol supervisors or certain officers to carry specific types of force equipment on duty, transport varying types of force equipment in their vehicle, or to have access to certain types of force equipment.

## Stage 4: Implementation of Risk Strategies

Implementing risk-control strategies consists of supervisors overseeing execution of the approach and enforcing that the strategy was correctly implemented. Supervisors play an important role in ensuring that the risk management control efforts are properly followed by line officers and need to shore up deficiencies as they emerge. Supervisors should also receive ongoing training commensurate with their duties, legality of their responsibilities, and in risk-control strategies. Moreover, they should be accessible in the field or cell block area on a regular basis, working along side officers in order to maintain an additional layer of agency and officer liability protection.

## Stage 5: Monitoring and Assessing Risk Control

Once risk-control strategies have been implemented, supervisory personnel should monitor the progress of application. When new policies, equipment, or a change in practice are adopted and implemented by officers, supervisors should monitor the application. This may be accomplished through varying methods: field observations, review of officer reports, tracking/analyzing use-of-force incidents, reviewing citizen/detainee complaints, review of incident videos, personnel evaluations, interviews of officers, and officer/supervisor training. Moreover, after a reasonable period of time, supervisors with officers should constructively evaluate the policy's implementation and/or incidents to determine the success or to assess problems that may have emerged since the implementation. With some regularity, departments institute a new policy, a new approach, or issue new equipment and fail to follow-up without field monitoring or evaluation. Assessment is necessary in order to determine what changes may be warranted and to determine future directions of the assessed strategy. Evaluating problems early can assist in proper decision making, making a change if necessary, assist in risk reduction, and reduce the potential of liability.

## Outcome

The net benefits of instituting such a risk management strategy, in regard to use-of-force issues with the population identified in this text include but are not limited to the following elements. First, the safety of officers can be enhanced through implementing risk management strategies. Second, applying risk-control strategies can improve employee performance and agency operations. Managing violent street-level and cell-block incidents where higher forms of force may be required and where multiple officers may have to respond can be enhanced. This can decrease the number of citizen complaints and detainee grievances. Third, performing an incident analysis can improve procedures and responses in circumstances where force is required. Incident analysis can also be useful in identifying the number of officers that should be deployed and in identifying the type of equipment needed for officers to employ when faced with a violent encounter. The analysis is most helpful in directing officers what to do prior to and after the restraint process.

Fourth, incident analysis can be useful in addressing the type of training that officers should be receive with regularity. This can increase officer and subject safety, enhance officer decision making, and direct officer and supervisory response to these incidents. Fifth, incorporating risk management techniques fulfills an administrative function. Administrators institute proactive management measures by implementing such strategies and enhance the organizational effectiveness. Sixth, risk management strategies place the department and personnel in the best defensible position against multiple claims of liability and/or potential misconduct. Hence, adopting a risk management approach to a high-profile/high-liability area, such as wrongful sudden in-custody deaths, can increase an organization's ability to control foreseeable risks, more efficiently direct employees in their job duties, and work toward reducing identifiable use of force risks. Adhering to sound risk management proactive principles is preferable to attempting to build a reactive defense after a sudden in-custody death has occurred. Implementing such a system can illustrate that the department and personnel have made a legitimate good faith effort to address an emerging problem consistent with reasonable management principles, legal standards, and professional practices.

## RESEARCH FINDINGS ON USE-OF-RESTRAINT POLICY AND TRAINING

In 1992, the San Diego Police Department's Task Force on Custodial Deaths *(9)* released its research findings regarding sudden in-custody deaths after a violent restraint incident. Responses were received from 145 police agencies representing 48 states. Respondents indicated incurring 94 restraint related in-custody deaths from 1969 to 1992. The responses revealed that 64% used some form of leg-restraint tool to control violent arrestees, 30% authorized the use of the hogtie procedure as necessary, 34% authorized the use of the carotid restraint as a force option, and 25% developed special needs procedures for dealing with suspects displaying bizarre or violent behavior. Of the respondents 62% felt confident in the methods used to transport a "maximally restrained" violent subject, 72% indicated that their defensive tactics training was adequate, that they routinely used the maximum restraint procedure with violent arrestees, and a plurality reported that they had used pain-compliance holds, physical strength techniques, and used body weight in a significant number of incidents to control and restrain persons. Based upon the findings of the survey task force members recommended policy, training and transport revisions for restrained violent arrestees.

A research project was conducted in 2004 to determine the current status of restraining violent arrestees or detainees in detention facilities *(10)*. Respondents to the surveys were defensive tactics instructors and/or administrators who were attending training seminars conducted by the researcher. The total number of responding agencies included 216 agencies from 29 states, which included municipal agencies (40%), sheriff departments (25%), correctional agencies (22%; prison/jail), and state police agencies (13%). Regions of the United States from which the respondents represented included north Atlantic (24%), central states (19%), south/southeast Atlantic (25%), and west (31%). Department size included (sworn officers) 50 to 100 officers (48%), 101–200 officers (27%), and 300-plus officers (25%). Only 10% of respondents reported experiencing a case of sudden in-custody death from 1990 through 2004. The death led to a lawsuit in 67% of cases; the agency prevailed in 48% of these cases, the plaintiff in 12%, and an out-of-court settlement was reached in the remaining 40% of cases.

Of respondents, 79% reported the existence of a policy that addressed authorized restraints (i.e., handcuffs, leg restraints, flex cuffs, belly chains, leg straps hobbles, straight jacket, restraint board, four-point restraint, and restraint chair), 88% did not allow the hogtying restraint method, 72% provided training in authorized restraints, and 40% provided annual training in the use of the authorized restraints. On average, however, 56% of the respondents revealed that the last time officers attended in-service training on the use of restraints was 3.5 years previously. Policy allowed transporting a maximally restrained subject in a police vehicle in 61% of the agencies. A policy statement on transporting a maximally restrained subject was contained in the policy in 60% of the policies and included three types of vehicles: patrol car (71%), ambulance (37%), and police van (18%).

Furthermore, 78% of respondents revealed that a policy existed for responding to the psychologically impaired, 68% had a policy for responding to subjects suspected of being under the influence of alcohol, and 65% percent had a policy for responding to suspects suspected of being under the influence of an illicit drug. The respondents reported that their department had provided special subject control technique training (62%), and multiple officer response training (57%). Although 49% had received training on responding to incidents involving the mentally impaired and those suspected of being under the influence in the previous 3 years, 51% had not received this training in more than 6 years.

Subject control technique training included control holds, take-down maneuvers, pressure points, neck restraint, swam method, tasers, cell extractions, impact weapon, and aerosols. On average, respondents revealed that they had received training within the previous 4 years specific to positional asphyxia (64%), in-custody deaths (50%), alcohol intoxication (48%), excited delirium (40%), and cocaine intoxication (38%).

These results reveal that a majority of agencies across the country have taken proactive steps to address the response of a violent restraint situation. Only 10% indicated that they had incurred an in-custody restraint death in the previous 14 years. Policy and training have been developed that instruct direct officer response in these confrontations. The findings showed that larger sized departments (>200 officers) are more likely to address these confrontations with policy, more frequent training, specific types of restraint equipment (i.e., handcuffs, hobble/leg straps), and directions for transporting a maximally restrained subject. The San Diego study revealed that 34% of the agencies allowed the use of the hogtied procedure, whereas only 12% in this study allowed officers to use the method. Litigated case outcomes reveal that 48% were settled and 40% were won by the defendant police agency, which shows the importance of providing sound policy, direction, and frequent training agency personnel.

## POLICY DEVELOPMENT RECOMMENDATIONS

An essential component of addressing sudden in-custody deaths in police or detention custody is the development of a use-of-force policy that directs officers in the appropriate response. It is important to underscore that each force encounter will obviously be different, comprising enumerable arrest or control variables. Officers cannot script their responses to a confrontation beforehand and the totality of the circumstances will direct the officer(s) degree of force and equipment that maybe employed. Therefore, the following components are recommended for consideration when contemplating policy revisions that can serve as a framework to guide officer decision making. The recommendations are also based on findings of above-cited research results and analysis of 225 use-of-force policies from police and detention agencies nationwide.

### Suggested Components of the Use-of-Force Policy

It is not the purpose here to recommend the specific written language of the policy because there are varying differences in jurisdictions and variations between sizes, purposes, and needs of departments, particularly between police agencies and detention facilities. Rather, the purpose here is to provide recommended components that should be considered in drafting such a policy. Recommendations are based on the need to use force, the dynamics of a violent use-of-force encounter (short of lethal force), the need for multiple officers to respond to violent restraint confrontations, the need to use higher degrees of force measures, and the need to use varying types of restraint equipment.

1. Policy statement: The first component of the policy should identify a statement that clearly describes the purpose and objectives of the policy. An additional statement may identify the response to "Special Needs Arrestees/Detainees."

2. Definitions: This section should identify varying elements requiring definitions and may include definitions of resistance, control, objectively reasonable force, less lethal force, lethal force, vehicles as lethal force, sudden in-custody death, restraint stress, and excited delirium.

3. Statutory and case law language: This section would comprise language that references state law, constitutional case holdings, and authority to use force. The *Graham v. Connor* (1989) case should be referenced in this section for police use-of-force issues comprised in accordance with the Fourth Amendment. In detention centers, reference should be made to the Fourteenth Amendment and the "Shocks the Conscience" standard in accordance to the *Johnson v. Glick* (1973) decision. Finally, prison personnel should reference the *Hudson v. McMillian* (1992) standard pertaining to using force in good faith to restore order and not for malicious purposes in accordance with the Eighth Amendment. This section should also address the parameters and the responsibility of using force measures.

4. Resistance categories: This section should identify and describe generic types of resistance officers may encounter. Types of resistance may include psychological intimidation, verbal and passive resistance, defensive resistance, active aggression, and deadly force types of resistance *(6)*.

5. Levels of officer force/control: This section should consist of descriptions of the options of officer control. This section could be divided into four subsections. First, less lethal force options should be identified, which include officer presence, verbal commands, and empty-hand control techniques. Second, the use of varying restraints should be addressed, including handcuffs, leg restraints, hobbles, leg straps/wraps, flex cuffs, belly chains, soft restraints, and the restraint chair. Third, intermediate weapons should be addressed, which could include aerosols, impact weapons, stun guns, less lethal projectiles, canines, and flashlights. Finally, lethal force options should be specified. The section should conclude with guidelines that direct officers when to consider using a level of force or a particular type of force equipment.

6. Team take-down control system: This section should comprise a discussion on the response of multiple officers. Generally, three to five officers respond to a violent restraint confrontation and a discussion of each officer's responsibility in taking a subject under control and restrain should be addressed. Team control techniques and the restraint process should be outlined as well as aftercare and follow-up procedures.

7. Variables affecting the use of force: Variables that should be addressed may include the number of subjects, officer reaction time, strength of the subject, age and size of the subject, environmental issues, rapidly evolving events, availability of back-up, and perception of the officer. The principles of escalation and de-escalation should be explained. As well, the principle of the totality of circumstances and the "One + One" theory should be addressed.

8. Response to a subject exhibiting bizarre behaviors: This section should outline the circumstances, behaviors, and response of officers who encounter a "violent and acting-out" subject. Considerations for control, restraint, medical care, and transport should be described.

9. Use-of-force for medical intervention: Detention/correctional agencies and police departments that maintain a lock-up should compose a section that describes the authorization for using force measures and equipment for medical/psychiatric intervention purposes. This may include situations in which a prisoner exhibits self-harming behaviors or requires medical care and has refused to cooperate with health care personnel or officers.

   Detention and lock-up personnel should also ensure that a thorough admission screening is conducted as the situation allows. If the detainee is cooperative during admission, a visual assessment should be performed and documented on a screening form. Medical care personnel should also perform a health care assessment within a reasonable period of time. It is advisable that one takes and documents the detainee's blood alcohol content. If the detainee is uncooperative or unable to undergo admission questioning because of his or her degree of inebriation or psychological state, personnel should monitor the individual until it is reasonable to conduct the questioning/assessment.

10. Monitoring a restrained subject: This section should address monitoring procedures of restrained subjects after a violent use-of-force encounter. This section should describe the subject's verbal, physical, physiological, and psychological behaviors/symptoms for officers to monitor. It should also detail when supervisory personnel should be summoned/notified. Statements, which direct officers in the proper decontamination procedures after the use of an aerosol, as well as after-care, should be addressed when a projectile, stun gun, canine, impact weapon, or a neck restraint are employed. Manufacturer protocols should be followed when employing any use-of-force equipment.

11. Medical considerations: This section should identify when an officer should consider rendering life-saving procedures and/or summoning emergency medical care personnel to the scene. In policing or in detention centers, when feasible, summoning medical care to the location or to a cell prior to the use-of-force incident should be considered.

12. Transportation procedures: This section should address how the restrained subject should be transported and in what type of vehicle. Each case will present different variables for officers to consider and the policy should allow for discretion in officer/supervisor decision making. If emergency medical care personnel transport the subject to the hospital, an officer should accompany them to the hospital and another officer should follow in a patrol unit. If officers transport the arrestee, a description of how the restrained subject is to be transported, the number of officers required for performing the transport, monitoring procedures to be used during transport, method of restraint, direction for considering transporting to a hospital, directions for transporting physically or mentally impaired persons, and

instructions to radio ahead to the hospital or detention center should be described. Special transport situations should also be included.

13. Reporting use of force: This section should explain that responding officers will submit a report indicating their participation in the incident. The report at a minimum should include the following:

   - A description of the nature of the incident.
   - An assessment and observations of the officers, including all behaviors, verbalization, and types of resistance offered by the subject.
   - A description of any weapons used by the subject.
   - Officer actions in the confrontation, including the number of officers who responded, calling for back-up/supervisors, verbal instructions used, physical control methods attempted/used, intermediate weapons attempted/used, lethal force measures used (if any).
   - The type of restraints that were used and how they were used.
   - Condition of the subject after restraint and monitoring procedures used after restraint.
   - First aid/life-saving techniques used by officers.
   - Summoning of emergency medical care personnel and their arrival.
   - Decontamination procedures used (if any).
   - Transportation procedures used (*see* Table 1 for the report checklist).

14. Investigation of force incidents: This section should describe the type of incidents that would trigger an internal or external investigation. It should also address responsibilities of involved officers and supervisors.

These 14 sections represent the suggested minimum sections contained in a policy that addresses the use of force and officers response. In developing and/or revising the force policy, administrators are encouraged to review state standards, professional standards, policies from other agencies, model policies, case law, legal department input, use-of-force training curriculum, use-of-force literature, and research literature on sudden in-custody deaths. Risk managers for the agency and the legal department should also be consulted.

Some departments may choose to address some of the sections of the suggested policy by developing separate policies on a particular topic. For example, an agency may wish to design a separate policy on transporting arrestees/detainees or high-risk incidents/arrests and address specific issues pertaining to the subject matter. Other departments may desire to develop a separate policy on responding to "violent special needs arrestees" and address the subject matter from this perspective. Furthermore, detention personnel may select to develop a specific policy that addresses use of force issues apart from street issues. For example, detention personnel may choose to design one policy that addresses use of force, another that describes forced cell extractions/insertions, a policy on confining and responding to prisoners exhibiting psychological

**Table 1**
**Checklist for Officer's Report in a Sudden In-Custody Death**

**Officer's Approach to the Incident**

- Dispatched
- Executing a warrant/commitment order
- Own initiative
- Back-up unit
- Conducting a security check

**Officer's Observation of the Subject**

- Bizarre behaviors (describe)
- Physical actions (specify)
- Appearance (hygiene, clothing/partial clothing, sweating)
- Injury(s) to the subject
- Skin color
- Verbal statements/threats made (shouting, etc.)
- Types of resistance and duration
- Response to officer's instructions
- Complaints made by the subject
- Hallucinations
- Influence of chemicals
- Strength of the subject
- Threshold to pain
- Combative to tranquil
- Possession/access to weapons

**Assessment on Location**

- Property damage
- Injuries to others
- Witnesses/relatives statements or interference
- Type of location (residence, hotel, street, business, cell, etc.)
- Confined space
- Lighting
- Location Hazards

**Officer's Actions**

- Initial assessment of subject
- Initial discussions with subject/others
- Verbal instructions with the subject
- Empty-hand control techniques used (specify)
- Aerosol used (specify)
- Intermediate weapons used (specify)
- Lethal force

*(Continued)*

**Table 1**
**(Continued)**

- Restraints used (specify)
- Summoned back-up
- Summoned a supervisor
- Summoned emergency medical personnel
- Specify type of participation in the incident
- Officer injuries and necessary treatment (specify)
- Length of time of struggle with officers

**Monitoring the Subject**

- Subject behaviors after restraint
- Subject struggle against restraints
- Subject comments after restraint
- Officers instructions during monitoring
- Officers actions while monitoring
- Position of subject in restraints
- Subject skin color
- Functional consciousness
- Subject injuries
- Signs of medical distress
- Summoning emergency medical personnel
- Emergency medical personnel actions
- Decontamination procedures employed
- Life saving procedures used by officers/others (specify)

**Transporting of Subject**

- Method of transport
- Type of vehicle
- How subject restrained
- Subject's behaviors during transport
- Specify officers who transported
- Subject's behaviors/statements during transport
- Location/length of transport
- Radioed in advance of transport
- Transport by emergency medical

impairment, another that outlines the use of the restraint chair or other restraints, after-care and medical care issues. There is no one best method to address the topic. The idea is to ensure that the subject matter is addressed and that officers and supervisors are provided a framework for deciding an appropriate response based upon the circumstances facing them. The policy should be distributed to all officers and periodic training should be provided.

## TRAINING CONSIDERATIONS

The training of criminal justice personnel is not a luxury. In *City of Canton v. Harris* (1989), the US Supreme Court held that a governmental entity could be held liable under federal Section 1983 legal actions for claims of failure to train when such failure amounts to deliberate indifference. This can include an administrator of a department who consciously chooses not to provide training to officers for a subject area and in failing to do so, results in a person's constitutional right being violated. Actionable cases must demonstrate that a lack of training constituted "official city policy," actually caused the injury to the person, and that the "known" subject matter was not addressed through training. The Court held that the key to imposing liability is if the existence of a pattern or history of incidents occurring within an agency with training left unattended by administrators in addressing the problem.

There has been some confusion about the standard the Court established in determining deliberate indifference in failure to train claims. The Court ruled that the focus of training must address recurring tasks that an officer may encounter. The degree of training required need only be adequate to address a particular matter. The Court further held that a department should evaluate its needs and allocate appropriate resources. Hence, officers should receive regularly scheduled training commensurate to their duties that they perform with ongoing frequency.

Providing regular training to officers fulfills the Court's holding in *Canton* and serves as a viable risk management strategy. It can be instrumental in enhancing officer performance, increasing skill proficiency, directing officer decision making, enhancing officer safety, reducing risks of the job, and defending lawsuits. Performing an incident analysis, as described in stage 1 of the risk management process, can be useful in determining the frequency of officers performing specific job tasks and the frequency of contacting varying types of arrestees or detainees. The analysis will also be beneficial in specifically addressing the training needs of the department. Using various force techniques, restraints, and other equipment is used with such regularity and with varying populations, that ongoing training should be provided for officers.

The following areas should be considered when contemplating what training to provide officers on the subject of sudden in-custody deaths.

1. Once the policy has been developed, officers should receive their own copies and subsequent training should be provided. As policies and procedures change, officers should be provided with training that addresses the changes.
2. Officers should receive ongoing training regarding their legal responsibility when using force. Case law and liability issues pertaining to the use of force, including

the case of *Graham v. Connor* (1989), individual Appellate Circuit Court decisions on the use of force, cases addressing sudden in-custody deaths, and training on the constitutional limits of using force should be provided.

3. Officers should receive a block of training that addresses responding to high-risk incidents and responding to subjects who are mentally impaired and/or who appear to be under the influence of a chemical substance. The basics of assessing behaviors and verbalization of these subjects should be provided. This can be helpful in assisting officers in determining the best course of action when dealing with this population. The purpose of this training is not to make officers "clinical experts," but rather to provide fundamental training in order to increase an officer's awareness of the types of common behaviors that often portray actions of these populations. Within this block or in a separate block of training, information that outlines taking the mentally impaired into custody in response to a voluntary or involuntary commitment order should be provided. In some jurisdictions, a lack of policy and training have existed that have been problematic for officers when tasked with this assignment. Issues of excessive force, misuse or misapplication of restraints, failing to follow a state's legal requirements, and wrongful deaths have emerged, necessitating periodic training.

4. Training should be provided that addresses topic areas surrounding sudden deaths in police custody. Subject matters may include behaviors associated with excited delirium, medical/psychological care issues, summoning of emergency medical care personnel, summoning of supervisors, rendering first aid, and transportation methods and locations of transport. It is also recommend that officers keep proficient in their certification of rendering first aid.

   Training that focuses on officer assessment of behaviors may include noting bizarre and agitated behaviors, purposeless actions, running from officers, violently resisting or attacking officers, shouting, exhibiting a high threshold to pain, nude, partially clothed, or disrobing, exhibiting extreme strength, hallucinations, actions or statements of paranoia, and quickly moving from combative to tranquil behavior. After restraining the person, officers should be trained to monitor the subject's condition by checking the pulse of the person and observing signs of medical distress, which may include respiratory distress, skin color changes, hyperventilation, shaking uncontrollably, loss of functional consciousness, signs of significant physical injury, incoherency, and altered mentation. Watching for these signs can assist the officer in making the proper health care decisions.

5. Training in the application of varying use-of-force measures should be provided. The training should address the use of verbal commands, empty-hand control techniques, the proper application of authorized restraints, intermediate weapons/equipment, and lethal force. Because multiple officers often respond to these violent confrontations, a team take-down control system should be taught so that a coordinated control strategy is applied *(7–9)*. Many of the sudden in-custody deaths have occurred shortly after a violent person has been restrained and/or while in restraints. Training should then be directed in the proper restraining methods,

use of authorized restraining equipment, and monitoring persons in restraints after a violent encounter.

Instructors should design scenario-based training that is supported by the Topic Integrated model (TIM) of training. This type of training is designed to apply contextual and skill-related knowledge to "realistic" job encounters. The training is entrenched in utilizing stimulus–response training principles that expose officers to applying physical skills under a stressful confrontation. TIM blends topics and techniques and provides "realistic" training for officers. For example, instructors could design a training scenario that places officers in a context of serving an involuntary commitment order filed by a family to have a member of the family placed in psychiatric facility. The scenario would be designed so that responding officers are forced to use force measures and restraint equipment in taking the person into custody, thus fulfilling the purpose of the training model (topic and techniques).

This type of scenario-based exercise provides realistic training and adheres to the *Canton* ruling, which holds that officers should receive realistic training to recurring encounters they face. Such training assists officers in many facets of the job, such as applying departmental policy, applying legal and technique decision making, practicing the proper use-of-force techniques and restraints, particularly under stress, applying skills in the environment in which officers will actually be responding, practicing the team take-down control system, making specific decisions regarding medical care transportation of the person, and providing a process of assessment of officer decision making and skill application. Role-players should be used and trained in advance of the scenario, protective gear used by all individuals in involved in the scenario, safety officers present to oversee the exercise, and the scenario should be videotaped and constructively assessed with the officers afterward.

6. Officers should be trained to the proper methods and vehicles for arrestee/detainee transport. Because some sudden in-custody deaths have occurred during transport, appropriate training should be designed to address this issue. This area contains numerous variables to consider and training should consist of the contents of the transportation policy, who will transport the person, the number of officers needed to transport, the location of the transport, the use of seat belts, special needs arrestees, and the type of vehicle that will be used. Training that addresses emergency medical personnel and transport should also be performed.

7. Administrators should provide training for supervisors relative to their responsibility in responding to an/or directing officers in the course of controlling and restraining an individual. Furthermore, training for departmental investigators should be conducted. Such training may include death investigations, use-of-force techniques, use-of-force equipment, applicable departmental policies, witness interview skills, use-of-force case law, officer conduct assessment and officer reports, medical documents and evaluations, and symptomologies associated with sudden in-custody deaths.

Although officer training provides an important ingredient in the proper application of using force and other associated topic areas, it will not prevent all sudden in-custody deaths from occurring. The health condition and drug abuse lifestyle may be the primary cause of death of those who have died after a violent restraint struggle with officers. The objective of training then is to provide reasonable methods, response options, and appropriate equipment to maximize the safety of the officers and subject; as well as increase skill proficiency, so that they can best respond to the unpredictable nature and the rapidly evolving circumstances they may face. Maintaining a commitment to training in this subject matter will assist officers in making justifiable decisions and directing them in appropriate responses.

## SUDDEN IN-CUSTODY DEATH INVESTIGATION CONSIDERATIONS

If an agency incurs a sudden in-custody death, members of that department should be prepared to respond to a myriad of questions and perform an investigation into the incident. Questions can range from what caused the death, whether the officers used excessive force and contributed to the death, to who ultimately should be held responsible for the death. These are not easily answered questions as a sudden in-custody deaths can contain enumerable variables. Therefore, a thorough incident investigation conducted by police personnel is highly recommended.

Police and detention agencies should develop or revise existing policies for conducting sudden in-custody death investigations. It may mean that an agency simply add additional sections to an existing policy that addresses death investigations generally.

1. The agency should evaluate its respective state's standards/law for conducting such an investigation. Differing states require certain protocols be followed and investigators should be aware of the requirements.
2. The chief administrator should conduct an internal investigation or consider having an external entity conduct the investigation. Again, state law should be referenced to determine the requirement. Allowing an external agency to perform the investigation can assist in defending claims allegations of a less than thorough investigation by internal investigators.
3. The policy should identify a person who has the responsibility of handling media questions, including press conferences/releases, and notifying the next of kin. This person should be trained in how to perform this assignment. Moreover, adhering to this practice will assist in maintaining control of the investigation and responding to questions and accusations that will be lodged against the department. An appropriate administrator should contact the agency's legal counsel and risk manager as soon as is reasonable. A briefing should be conducted and all documentation

should be provided to counsel and the risk manager. As the investigation proceeds, periodic briefings should be held with these individuals to keep them abreast of the progress of the case.

4. Once it is learned that a sudden in-custody death has occurred, officers should advise that a supervisor and investigators are needed (if not already notified) and mark-off the scene and protect it so that investigators can perform an adequate and thorough investigation. Investigators should arrive on the scene and receive a briefing relative to the nature of the incident. A walk through of the scene should be conducted paying attention to scene boundaries, entry and exit points, and location of evidence. Investigators should begin taking photos of the scene, decedent (if still on location), and restraints and force devices used. Investigators should also videotape the scene, collect/inventory and safeguard evidence, and record scene item measurements. Interviews should be conducted and statements taken from emergency medical personnel involved in the incident, attending hospital physicians involved in the care of the decedent, and other witnesses to the event *(10–12)*. Investigators may consider making a re-enactment of the incident and videotaping it.

On-scene investigators should record the climatic conditions of the incident and time of day. All environmental variables should be described and noted. Descriptions of the condition and location of the scene should be noted (i.e., street, field, house, alleyway, dimensions of a room, temperature, ice, snow, water, number of persons present, day/night, etc.). In interviewing civilian witnesses, investigators can obtain pertinent information regarding the decedent's behaviors or activities in the preceding hours, days, or weeks prior to police contact. This can be most helpful in obtaining a complete assessment of the subject prior to police intervention.

5. Involved officers should submit reports within a reasonable period of time and should be allowed to submit a supplemental report after completion of one or two sleep cycles *(7,14,15)*. Officer interviews should be conducted after completing a sleep cycle and in accordance to constitutional rights under *Garrity v. New Jersey* (1979), union contract, and departmental policy. In accordance with departmental policy, involved officers may be placed on administrative leave pending the investigation. Supervisory personnel summoned to the scene or the shift supervisor should also submit a report and be interviewed by investigators.

6. Investigators should retain all radio communication recordings made between dispatch, officers, and individuals who may have summoned the police. Any car camera videos and/or closed-circuit videos taken in a detention facility should be retained, preserved, and reviewed. Other videos that may have been made by surveillance cameras or witnesses should be retained and reviewed.

7. An investigator should compile a file on the incident. Contents may comprise officer reports, interviews, witness interviews/statements, relevant policies, training/personnel files of the involved officers/supervisors, inventory of evidence, photos, drawings, a time line of the sequence of the events, property, videos of TV coverage/press conferences, newspaper articles, emergency medical personnel's report/statements, attending hospital physician's report/statement, notification of the next of kin, reports, and subject information. The file may expand during the

investigation and the investigator should ensure the safekeeping of the contents of the file. Items within the file should be itemized, numbered, and safely filed in a notebook/binder *(16–18)*. Throughout the investigation, the investigators should keep the appropriate commander appraised as to the progress of the investigation and document such progress reports.

8. An investigator or assigned individual from the department should attend the autopsy as this is of paramount importance. Photos should be taken of the body prior to, during, and after the autopsy. An interview of the attending pathologist and/or medical examiner should be conducted regarding possible causes of death. The agency investigator should request a toxicology, histology, and serology analysis be performed on the decedent. Do not assume that these three assessments will automatically be performed. Toxicology will identify any chemical substances in the body, while histology reveals the condition of the tissue of the body, and serology reveals the condition of the blood in the body.

Once the autopsy and other medical reports have been completed an investigator should receive and assess the causes and manner of death and findings of the report. Investigators are encouraged to pay attention to the toxicology, histology, and serology reports, the conditions of the internal organs, such as the size of the heart, whether the heart is diseased, size of the lungs, condition of the brain, kidneys, liver, thyroid, and spleen, needle marks/tracks on the arms or legs, marks/bruising on the body, artifacts that occurred after the death or time of the autopsy, and signs of life saving efforts on the body (i.e., bruised/broken sternum/ribs, abrasions, pectichae in the eyes/scalp).

9. Investigators should conduct an extensive investigation into the background of the decedent *(19–23)*. The investigation should include the following important areas: family history, residential history, employment history, military history, medical/psychiatric history, arrest/conviction history, incarceration history, behavioral history, and substance abuse history. Acquiring a complete history of the decedent can provide additional information regarding his or her background that may be useful in more completely understanding a cause of sudden death that may be problematic when a negative autopsy is determined.

10. Once the investigation is complete, the investigator should submit a detailed and thorough report. The report documents how the investigation was conducted, and should the following items: identification of all officers involved, witness statements and interviews, all reports reviewed, evidence collected/processed, all photos taken, videos and diagrams created, tests performed if any, measurements made, dispatch tapes, all interviews and statements taken of police and medical personnel, securing/processing of equipment used by officers, medical history of decedent, relevant policies of the agency, legal assessments made by the prosecutor, and other documents reviewed during the investigation. The investigator's report should only report the findings of the investigation and not include his or her recommendations. The report should then be submitted to the proper administrator in the department for his or her review. A checklist for investigators is contained in Table 2.

### Table 2
### Investigators Checklist

**On scene**
- Scene briefing
- Scene walk through
- Photographs, measurements, drawings, videos
- Collecting/securing evidence
- Officer statements/interviews
- Witness interviews/statements
- Environmental conditions
- Follow laws of collecting evidence

**File**
- List of evidence
- Storage of evidence
- List of witnesses/statements/interviews
- List of officers/statements
- Officer interviews
- Officers reports
- Appropriate policies
- Use-of-force training
- List of force equipment used
- Create time line of events
- Officer reports
- Emergency medical personnel reports (on scene/at hospital)
- Autopsy report
- Toxicology, histology, and serology reports
- Media coverage
- Communication tapes
- Shift logs
- Re-creation of incident/video produced
- Prosecutor's evaluation/report
- Running documentation of the progress of the investigation

**Decedent History**
- Family
- Residential
- Employment
- Military
- Educational
- Substance abuse
- Medical

*(Continued)*

**Table 2**
**(Continued)**

- Psychological
- Nutritional
- Arrest/convictions
- Incarceration

**Police Intervention**

- Nature of contact
- Behaviors/statements of the decedent
- Actions of the decedent
- Officers verbal instructions
- Officers use of empty-hand control techniques
- Officers use of aerosols
- Officers use of intermediate weapons
- Officers use of lethal force
- Officers use of restraints
- Officers summon supervisors/investigators
- Position of decedent after restraint
- Behaviors of decedent after restraint
- Decontaminate procedures used
- First aid rendered by officers
- Officers summon emergency medical care
- Monitoring restrained subject by officers

**Medical Care Personnel**

- How summoned to scene
- Time of arrival/departure of emergency medical on scene
- Assessment made by medical care
- Actions of emergency medical on scene
- Medical care provided

**Transport**

- Police vehicle
- Medical vehicle
- Location/length of transport
- Transported in restraints
- Position in vehicle
- Number of officers in police transport
- Officers monitor subject during transport
- Decedent behaviors/statements during transport
- Medical care rendered during transport

*(Continued)*

**Table 2**
***(Continued)***

**Hospital Care**
- Behaviors/statements of subject at hospital
- Medical care administered
- Attending health care workers
- Length at hospital
- Interview/statements of health care personnel
- Reports of attending health care personnel

**Autopsy**
- When performed
- Performed by
- Who attended
- Photo's taken
- Autopsy report
- Toxicology report
- Histology report
- Serology report
- Cause of death
- Manner of death

## OTHER CONSIDERATIONS

### Critical Incident Debriefing

Within in a reasonable period of time, an incident debriefing should be conducted. A post-incident team comprised of trained individuals to deal with the potential psychological issues experienced by involved officers should be developed prior to the incident. The purpose is to provide a structured period of debriefing for involved officers to discuss their feelings and emotions to trained personnel. Agency administrators should not be part of this process. Referrals to employee assistance programs should be made to officers who desire further counseling or who do not feel comfortable in participating in the critical debriefing session.

### Final Incident Review

Administrators should conduct a final incident review and critique once the investigation is completed. The purpose of the meeting is not to engage in finger-pointing or fault-finding, but to constructively assess the incident and response in order to work toward reducing the likelihood of further such incidents if feasible. Officers, supervisors, trainers, medical personnel, investigators, and other appropriate personnel should be involved in the assessment review. Recommendations should be made and documented as warranted; and efforts made to make the necessary changes as needed. Detention facilities should report all custodial deaths in compliance with the Custody Reporting Act of 2000 (no. 106-297) to the Department of Justice.

## CONCLUSIONS

A sudden in-custody death involves a milieu of complex factors. As members of society continue to lead unhealthy lifestyles through abusing drugs and as police contacts continue with the mentally impaired, the likelihood that an in-custody death may occur continues to present problems for police, medical, and legal professions, as well as for society in general. Therefore, administrators, officers, trainers, and health care workers are encouraged to continue to be prepared in their response to these situations by developing workable policies, providing training for officers in reasonable responses, and conducting thorough and complete investigations. Striving to incorporate the suggestions described here can assist in that preparation.

## REFERENCES

1. Ross DL. Assessing in-custody deaths in jails. American Jails 2001;Nov–Dec: 13–25.
2. Ross DL. Civil Liability in Criminal Justice (3rd ed.). Anderson Publishing, Cincinnati, OH, 2003.
3. Ball J, Kissin W. The DAWN report: trends in drug-related emergency department visits, 1994–2001. Office of Applied Studies Abuse and Mental Health Services Administration, Rockville, MD, 2003 pp. 1–8.
4. Guy E, Platt J, Zwerling I, Bullock S. Mental health status of prisoners in an urban jail. Crim Justice Behav 1985;1:29–53.
5. Steadman HS, Fabisiak S, Dvoskin J, Holohean E. A survey of mental disability among state prison inmates. Hosp Community Psychiatry 1989;1: 1086–1089.
6. Teplin LA. The prevalence of sever mental disorder among male urban jail detainees: Comparison with the eipdemiologic catchment area program. Am J Public Health 1990;6:663–669.
7. Beck AJ, Maruschak LM. Mental health treatment in state prisons, 2000. U.S. Department of Justice, Bureau of Justice Statistics, Washington, DC, 2001.
8. Siddle BK. Defensive tactics instructor manual. Pressure Point Control Tactics, Management Systems, Bellville, IL, 1996.
9. Krosch C, Binkard V, Blackbourne B. Final report of the custody death task force. San Diego, California Police Department, San Diego, 1992.

10. Ross DL. An analysis of restraint policies and training. Unpublished technical report, East Carolina University, Greenville, NC, 2005.
11. Ross DL, Siddle BK. An analysis of the effects of survival stress in police use of force encounters. Law Enforcement Exec Forum J 2003;3: 9–26.
12. Klugiewicz G. The star tactic: a five officer takedown. The Law Enforcement Trainer 2000;15:28–31.
13. Albrecht JF. The Restraint Report: The Task Force on the Restraint of Suspects Who Resist Arrest in New York. New York City Police Department, New York, NY, 1994.
14. Clark SC. National Guidelines for Death Investigation: Research Report. US Department of Justice, Washington, DC, 1997.
15. Rau RM. Crime Scene Investigation. US Department of Justice, Washington, DC, 2000.
16. Eliopulos LN. Death Investigator's Handbook: A Field Guide to Crime Scene Processing, Forensic Evaluations, and Investigative Techniques. Paldin Press, Boulder, CO, 1993.
17. Siddle BK. Sharpening the Warrior's Edge. PPCT Research Publications, Millstadt, IL.
18. Grossman D, Siddle BK. Critical Incident Amnesia: The Physiological and Psychological Basis and Implications of Memory Loss During Extreme Survival Stress Situations. PPCT Management Systems, Millstadt, IL, 1998.
19. Copeland AR. Deaths in custody revisited. Am J Forensic Med Pathol 1984;2:121–124.
20. Eckert G. Medicolegal investigation of problems involving criminals and criminal activity. Am J Forensic Med Pathol 1983;3: 279–286.
21. Shull TJ. Custody death: managing the crisis from investigation to litigation. American Jails 2001;Nov–Dec:38–47.
22. Di Maio DJ, Di Maio VJM. Forensic Pathology. Elsevier, New York, NY, 1989.
23. Lawerence C. Investigator protocol: Sudden in-custody death. Police Chief 2004;1:25–31.

## CASES CITED

*City of Canton Ohio v. Harris*, 489 U.S. 378 (1989)
*Graham v. Connor*, 490 U.S. 386 (1989)
*Hudson v. McMillian*, 503 U.S. 1 (1992)
*Johnson v. Glick*, 481 F.2d 1028 (2nd Cir. 1973)
*Monell v. New York City of Department of Social Services*, 436 U.S. 658 (1978)

# Index